THE BEGINNING INVESTOR

Second Edition

A Medical Economics Book

THE BEGINNING INVESTOR

Second Edition

Philip Harsham

Medical Economics Books
Oradell, New Jersey 07649

Library of Congress Cataloging in Publication Data
Harsham, Philip.
   The beginning investor.

   Rev. ed. of: The beginning investor / edited by
Bernard J. Hassan. c1982.
   Bibliography: p.
   Includes index.
   1. Investments—Addresses, essays, lectures.
2. Tax shelters—Addresses, essays, lectures.
3. Physicians—Finance, Personal—Addresses, essays,
lectures. I. Title.
HG4522.H37   1983   332.6'78   83-13459
ISBN 0-87489-365-8

ISBN 0-87489-365-8
Medical Economics Company Inc.
Oradell, New Jersey 07649
   First Edition   February 1982
   Second Edition   January 1984

Printed in the United States of America

Copyright © 1984 by Medical Economics Company Inc., Oradell, N.J. 07649. All rights reserved. None of the content of this publication may be reproduced, stored in a retrieval system, or transmitted in any form or by any means (electronic, mechanical, photocopying, recording, or otherwise) without the prior written permission of the publisher.

Contents

Publisher's preface **vi**

1. Introduction **1**
2. Taking the mystery out of the stock market **5**
3. Getting started in the bond market **25**
4. Picking a path through the mutual-fund maze **43**
5. Making the most out of the money market **57**
6. Tiptoeing profitably into real estate **71**
7. Some offers you *can* refuse **87**
8. Tax shelters: Looking before you leap **97**
9. Tax shelters: Playing to win in a risky game **109**
10. Further reading **127**

    Index **135**

Publisher's preface

Just about any financial adviser, competent or not, can come up with a few cutting remarks about the financial savvy of physicians. Probably one of the kinder ones goes like this: "If there's any group of investors more financially stupid than doctors, it's lawyers."

Well, we of course know some lawyers who are financially stupid. And some doctors, too. We even know some engineers, and salesmen, and computer wizards. Even some publishers.

That's by way of saying that this book has a past. Conceived by Philip Harsham, much of it was published originally as a series of articles he wrote for MEDICAL ECONOMICS magazine from 1979-80. The intent then was to give physicians, whose years of study had sidestepped all things financial, a little help in the game of investment "catch-up" so many of them seemed to be playing.

The articles proved so popular that we commissioned a free-lance editor, Bernard J. Hassan, to put them in book form. Published in 1982 as *The Beginning Investor*, the Hassan edition surpassed our own high expectations for it. Doctors bought it; lawyers bought it—we'd like to think that even a few financial advisers bought it (while wearing disguises, of course). In short, it was a sellout.

Now we're back with a second edition, this one updated, edited, and extensively rewritten to reflect the changes inevitable in a fast-moving investment climate.

If you're a beginning investor, you should find its plain-talk material very helpful. If you're a seasoned investor, value its plain talk and simplified explanations as rarities in the financial-writing field. And try not to be put off by the title; you can always hide it behind your *Wall Street Journal*.

About the author: Many physician readers of *The Beginning Investor* will recognize the author's byline. It has been appearing over financially oriented articles in MEDICAL ECONOMICS since 1965. Philip Harsham has become respected over those years as a writer who is adept at making complex financial subjects intelligible to the financially unsophisticated.

But Harsham, whose work has appeared in numerous other publications as well, often speaks of his "previous life"—his life as a newspaperman—when his presidency of a newsroom investment club at *The Louisville Courier-Journal* provided his closest contact with the financial world. His primary interest in that life was African affairs, an interest punctuated by extended tours of the African continent as a newsman and as a consultant on the African press to the Rockefeller Foundation.

Harsham moved to MEDICAL ECONOMICS from the foreign desk of *The New York Times*. Since 1970, he's served from a Florida base as MEDICAL ECONOMICS' Southeast editor. He and his wife Diane have two sons. The younger, Stephen, is studying computer engineering at Tulane University, where Harsham completed his undergraduate work. The elder, Douglas, was graduated last summer from Vanderbilt University and has entered, of all things, the investment field.

Introduction

1

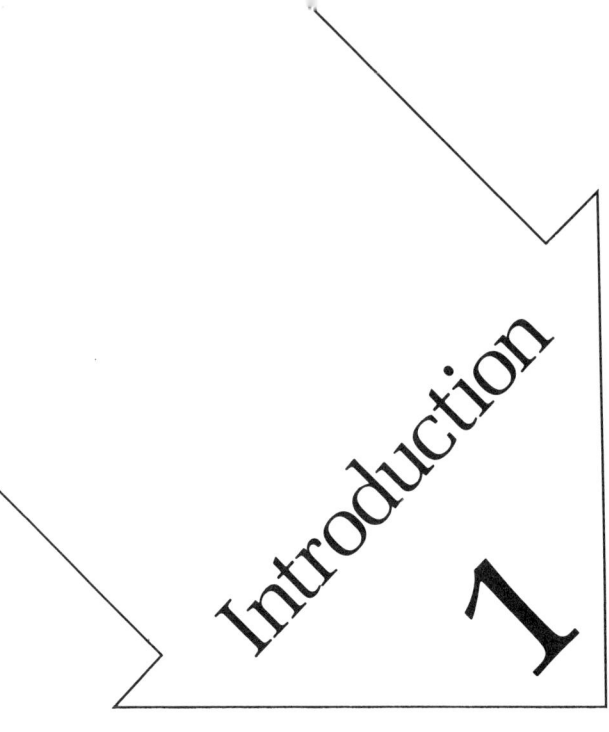

Introduction 1

A high level of income does not necessarily a wealthy man make. Not long ago, for example, a lawyer specializing in finance surveyed the personal finances of 150 top corporation executives and found that not one of them had done a satisfactory job of managing his own money.

That prompts a rather disturbing thought: If executives responsible for millions and billions in corporate funds fall short in managing their own finances, what should be expected of physicians whose formal training typically is bereft of financial studies?

The answer that follows naturally, of course, is "not much." Yet, as you hardly need to be told, physicians as a group form one of the more affluent segments of our society. Even the mean stipend of a third-year resident —$21,378 annually—is just about twice the per capita income for Americans in general; in fact, it exceeds the annual income of 88 percent of the nation's nongovernmental work force. (It should come as no surprise that 36 percent of government workers earn more than $25,000.)

It might well follow just as naturally, then, that the physician—indeed, any successful professional—needs to know something about money management, and especially about investing—if only to understand what a hired money manager or investment counselor is doing in his behalf.

That's the rationale behind this book. Contained herein is information for the intelligent, sophisticated earner who just happens to be unschooled, at least formally, in matters of finance.

Some of you may protest that parts of the book are too basic, perhaps an affront to your intelligence. But just as many may complain that it is at times too esoteric, assuming far greater investment knowledge on your part than it should.

Satisfying both the knowledgeable and the not-so-knowledgeable is the impossible task that confronts any writer who strives to serve a broad spectrum of readers. So we must ask that you approach *The Beginning Investor* much as you would a buffet table: Recognize it as a generous offering, but take from it only what your appetite calls for.

Even that approach demands an up-front cautionary note: Don't rush into an investment program. Invest only after you've formulated an investment plan—and once you've begun to invest, give that plan a checkup at least once a year to make sure it still conforms to your financial needs.

How do you formulate an investment plan? For starters, it's good to determine just how much you're actually worth. If you're a MEDICAL ECONOMICS reader, that's made easy for you via a worksheet the magazine publishes each November in its annual financial-planning issue. But you can come up with a workable figure simply by subtracting your total liabilities from your total assets.

That means totting up what you have in bank accounts, in life-insurance cash value, in equity in your home and other real-estate holdings, and in accounts receivable—all assets that have the potential for conversion into cash.

From that total deduct amounts you owe, including such things as insurance premiums and taxes that must be paid before the year's out. The result is your net worth.

For it to be very meaningful to you, you'll need to refer to your previous year's records and come up with a comparable computation for that year. By comparing the figures for the two years, you'll get a rough idea of how well—or how badly—your net worth (independent of your income) has grown.

Chances are, unless you've included some form of investment, your net worth's growth hasn't kept pace with inflation. If that's the case, of course, it's actually registered a loss.

That's where an investment plan comes in. You can design your plan to speed your net worth's growth toward a retirement goal. You can design it to give you more current income. You can design it to shelter investable income from taxes, thereby maximizing growth via tax-free compounding. These pages will help you think through your own needs and decide how they might best be met.

Bear in mind that the book aims to address, and inform, the beginning investor. If your investment expertise lifts you beyond that category, fine; you'll have no trouble finding a beginner to pass the book along to—there's a new crop of them every year.

Taking the mystery out of the stock market

2

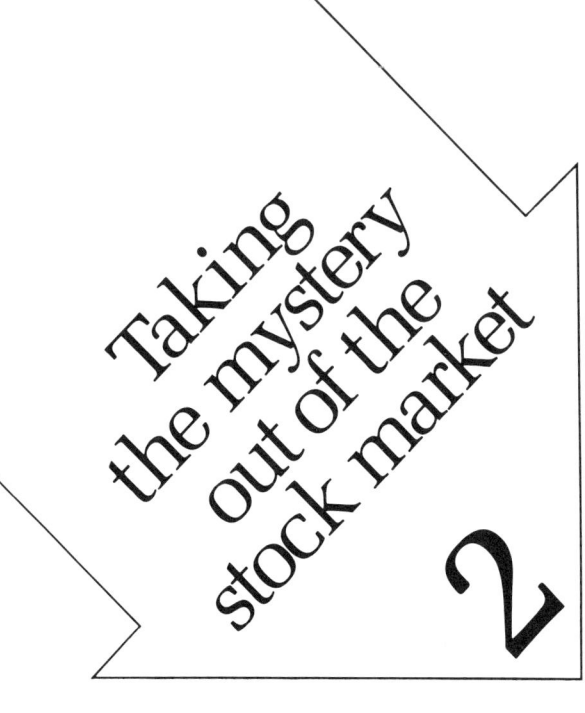

2. Taking the mystery out of the stock market

You have a steady and growing income, ample funds set aside for house payments and life insurance, and savings to see you through an emergency. Now you want to make your money earn more money, or you want to preserve your buying power in an inflationary economy. You may feel that you are ready to start investing your money in the stock market.

The first thing to do is forget that you ever heard the phrase "playing the market." Investing is not play. It's serious business, buying bits of equity in American industry. It's a business in which gains and losses occur continually, which means it's not the place for you if you can't abide daily ups and downs in your investment fortunes. It involves taking risks, but those risks should decrease in proportion to your investment knowledge. And it's the arena in which you can best cope with income tax laws that can scoop a lot of cream off the top of an investment's yield. That last point brings up the first major decision a stock investor must make.

INCOME OR CAPITAL GAINS?

If you're a younger physician, one who can expect at least 10 more years of high earnings from your profession, you should lean toward investing for capital gains—in other words, for growth. On the other hand, if you're beginning to plan for your retirement, or if you need to supplement your practice income, you would probably do better to concentrate on high-yield—or income—stocks.

Here's why:

1. So-called "growth" companies typically pay small dividends, or none at all, on their stock. Instead, they reinvest their profits, believing that money spent for research or new equipment will enhance future profits, attract investors, and run up the market price of their stock. In theory, then, a growth-stock investor forgoes immediate dividends in favor of a possibly much larger future profit—or capital gain—when he eventually sells his stock. The capital gain, of course, will be taxed at more favorable rates than dividends would be.

Say, for example, that you bought 100 shares of Walt Disney Productions in 1969 at 78 ($78 a share), when it was paying a cash dividend of only 7.5 cents a share each quarter. You would have invested $7,800, disregarding brokerage fees, with the prospect of earning only $30 in cash on it each year—a yield of less than 0.4 percent.

But let's say that you held on to Disney for 10 years. Your 100 shares would have grown through stock splits and extra dividends paid in stock to about 480 shares, worth roughly $16,500 in the 10th year. Your cash dividends, meanwhile, would have increased to 12 cents quarterly on each current share.

Now, to put all that in perspective: Even with the increased dividend, you'd be receiving a yield of only 1.4 percent—$230 in cash each year from an investment valued at $16,500. That "unearned" income can be taxed at the maximum rate, but the amount is small enough to pose little problem at income tax time.

Suppose, though, you chose to sell your stock. You'd have a capital gain of $8,700—112 percent over the 10 years, or an average of 11.2 percent annually. That would give you a total return of almost 13 percent annually (11.2 percent capital gains plus 1.4 percent dividends). Only the small dividend income would be fully subject to income taxes. Your $8,700 is a long-term capital gain, and as such it can be taxed at no more than 20 percent.

2. "Income" stocks lie at the opposite end of the spectrum. They usually represent companies with limited ability to expand or increase their earnings, so they must pay high dividends to attract investors. Those dividends are fully taxable as "unearned" ordinary income.

For an example, let's use Tenneco—a multifaceted conglomerate that traces its roots to the natural-gas transmission industry. Say you bought 100 shares of Tenneco in 1969, when it was selling at 27 and paying 32 cents a share in dividends every three months. You'd have been drawing a 4.7 percent annual yield.

At midyear 1979, you'd still have owned only 100 shares of Tenneco, and your $2,700 investment would have grown in value to only $3,500. That's a 3 percent average annual gain, hardly awe-inspiring in a decade characterized by double-digit inflation. But your quarterly dividend over those 10 years would have increased gradually to 55 cents a share—$2.20 a year—for an annual yield of almost 6.3 percent.

Your total return would come to 9.3 percent (3 percent capital gain plus 6.3 percent dividend). Not bad—until you consider that income taxes in the top bracket would almost halve your dividend income.

Investing in income stocks makes little sense, then, for the physician whose practice income is high. However, it's a sound way to provide income in your retirement, when your tax bracket will be less onerous. Balancing your portfolio with some good income stocks can also limit your risk of loss in a weak market. Their yields assure at least some degree of price stability. In contrast, growth stocks have little more than the potential of capital gains to recommend them. When untoward market conditions weaken investor confidence, growth stocks tend to drop in price much further—albeit they usually rebound faster—than income stocks.

In periods of high interest rates, such as the early 1980s, even growth companies must pay relatively high dividends to attract buyers for their shares. Companies that are maturing to the point where their growth rate has begun to level off tend to add a dividend "sweetener," too. International Business Machines is a classic example. In 1969, when high-flying IBM was selling at 42 times earnings, its dividend was a meager 1.2 percent. More recently, however, when it sold at 15 times its per-share earnings, it paid 3.1 percent, and a dividend increase was anticipated. Once synonymous with the term "growth stock," IBM is now held by some investors for both its growth and income propensities.

WHAT'S THAT STOCK WORTH?

We've just tossed in the term "per-share earnings," and it's a significant one. Corporations speak of their profits as earnings on invested capital. And because their capital is provided by investors, or shareholders, they commonly express their profits as earnings per share—i.e., the amount of earnings attributable to each share of stock outstanding.

Not surprisingly, per-share earnings become a measure of a stock's worth. But of two stocks earning $1 per share, one might sell for $10 a share while another might sell for $25. To put those earnings in focus, you use what's called the price-to-earnings ratio or, more commonly, the P/E. You arrive at it by dividing a stock's per-share price by its annual per-share earnings. So the $10 stock earning $1 has a P/E of 10, and the $25 stock has a P/E of 25.

All things being equal, the $10 stock is obviously the better buy, but in stocks all things seldom are equal. IBM, for example, was an excellent buy in 1969 at that price of 42 times earnings (a P/E of 42). At the same time, Cincinnati Gas & Electric was an excellent buy at 13 times earnings. It's a matter of comparing *similar* stock issues. IBM in 1969 still was the darling of growth stocks, and go-go investors were willing to bet heavily on its future earnings growth. Cincinnati G&E was typical of capital-intensive utilities, companies that must spend continually to meet the needs of expanding service areas. Like utilities in general, it had little earnings-growth potential to offer because state regulation of rates limited its profit margin.

P/E ratios, then, must be judged within their own milieu. IBM at a P/E of 42 would be more accurately weighed against Burroughs, which carried a P/E of 49 in that same period. And Cincinnati G&E's P/E of 13 could well have been edged out in the eyes of some investors by Pacific Lighting, with a P/E of 12.

While the P/E ratio provides a basic measure of a stock's relative worth, other factors are equally important. Perhaps a company has developed some new important technology—Texas Instruments and its semiconductors, for example. Perhaps it's taken a commanding lead in a difficult-to-penetrate industry, such as Schlumberger's in the oil-well services field. Or perhaps, like Albertson's in the supermarket field, it's scored an enviable progression of earnings increases. Then savvy investors take note, their buying catches the eye of less savvy investors, the number of shares changing hands balloons, and the stock's price takes off. (Unfortunately, it's only at this point that the beginning investor typically wakes up to a stock's potential—and catches it at its high.)

In truth, a stock is worth whatever the give-and-take of the market says it's worth. You can use its P/E ratio as a guide. You can weigh its market price against its book value, the total value of its intrinsic holdings. You can consider the size of the dividend it pays. The market—meaning the buying and selling of all investors combined—considers those things, too. Then it adds in such elements as investor psychology (shaped by economic and political developments, among other things), the stresses of supply and demand, and the gossip among Wall Street insiders. Those additives often have a greater effect on the price of a stock than any consideration of intrinsic values.

GETTING TO KNOW STOCKS

Anybody who's been exposed to high-school economics knows that there are actually two kinds of stocks—preferred and common.

Preferred stocks carry fixed dividends that must be paid ahead of any common-stock dividends, and holders of preferreds get first crack, after creditors and bondholders, at any assets left in the event the corporation has to liquidate. Preferreds accord shareholders preferential treatment, but individual investors who might opt for preferreds find that bonds and other fixed-income instruments are better paying and more interesting these days. As a result, preferreds aren't much traded.

That's not always the case, however, as the early 1983 market demonstrated. With interest rates in general slipping downward, investors who'd become accustomed to high yields from other investments were reluctant to accept lesser amounts. Many discovered high-yielding preferreds playing wallflower, simply passed over by investors attuned to sexier numbers.

The more savvy among them began picking up preferreds that paid fixed yields of 14, 15, and 16 percent, while returns on more glamorous investments were hitting the 8 percent level. The stepped-up trading had prices of preferreds yo-yoing in a most atypical manner.

You'll hear more about this anomaly in investor thinking in a later chapter. Just accept the fact that, for the most part, preferreds are relatively little traded. We'll concentrate, therefore, on common stocks, so named because they represent shares in companies that are owned in common by stockholders.

Listed stocks are traded on the New York Stock Exchange (NYSE), the American Stock Exchange (ASE), and several regional exchanges. Unlisted stocks, usually stocks of smaller companies that have not yet met the prerequisites for exchange listing, are traded in the over-the-counter (OTC) market. This OTC trading activity is monitored daily by the National Association of Securities Dealers. Price quotations are made available to news media, but not the more complete composite report that is given for trading in listed stocks.

Probably your best way to gain familiarity with stocks and what they're doing is to become a conscientious reader of your paper's business pages. If your local paper falls short in market coverage (and most of them do), turn to The Wall Street Journal ($94 a year, delivered). The Journal's satellite-transmitted editions make same-day delivery possible in a growing number of cities.

If you're seriously considering a stock for purchase, you should, of course, know more about it than newspaper listings can teach you. You'll want to research the issuing corporation as well as the stock's past actions, using reference materials compiled and updated by

Standard & Poor's, Moody's, Value Line, and a few specialized services. You should find most everything you need in the reference departments of stock-brokerage offices. Better public libraries offer at least some Moody's and Standard & Poor's publications, as well as *Barron's*, a weekly Dow Jones publication that gives a comprehensive rundown on market activities. Box 2-1 summarizes the kinds of information you should look for.

FINDING A STOCKBROKER

You'll have no trouble finding a stockbroker; the more aggressive ones will find you. The trick is to find a broker you'll want to deal with.

The late Gerald Loeb, one of the most successful brokers of all time, liked to make his position clear with clients: "You don't have to like me, and I don't have to like you. But if you're going to trust me to invest your money, we at least have to respect each other."

To find a broker you can respect, do what your patients do when they're looking for a family doctor—ask among knowledgeable friends. Or seek recommendations from your bank or accountant. Or walk into a brokerage office—Box 2-2 on page 16 lists some top firms—and take your chances.

If you do become a "walk-in," at least start with the office manager. Give him some idea of your investment objectives, and let him put you with the broker he thinks might be best for you. Otherwise, a receptionist will lead you to the broker who's least busy at the moment—and there's usually a good reason why he's least busy.

At the very least, you need a broker to place your orders to buy and sell stock. At the most, you may give him full discretion to choose the stocks for your portfolio, and to decide when he'll purchase them for you and how long they'll be held.

You should expect him to stay abreast of developments affecting stocks of interest to you and alert you to advantageous buying and selling opportunities. Of course, he and his firm should provide you with a complete and prompt accounting of all your transactions. But if you let him know that you consider him an order taker only, you shouldn't be surprised if you hear very little from him.

You'd be wise to stick with full-service brokers, at least until you've gained confidence in your own ability to research stocks. Visit the broker's office, make use of

BOX 2-1

What you'll find in a good

The quality of financial reporting varies widely among newspapers. Here are the basic items of information that any investor should look for:

▶ *The gain or loss* in the Dow Jones Industrial Average (DJIA), the most widely used barometer of stock market activity, and perhaps changes in the Standard & Poor's and New York Stock Exchange indices as well. These readily indicate market direction. A report that "the market gained 3 points today" might mean, for instance, that the DJIA (made up of 30 selected common stocks) rose from yesterday's market close of 1205 to close today at 1208.

▶ *The high* that each stock's price reached during the day's trading, **the low, the closing price,** and **the net change** from the previous day's close to the present day's close.

▶ *The trading range* for each stock over the last 52 weeks. That's the highest price paid for an issue during the period and the lowest—information that helps you place the current price in perspective.

his firm's reference materials, let him get to know you. You'll each do well to learn how the other thinks.

Once you feel competent enough to manage your own stock portfolio, you may want to investigate the discount brokerage houses. While full-service brokerage firms maintain expensive research staffs and provide a goodly amount of handholding, most discounters do nothing more than execute buy and sell orders. Their appeal is lower commissions. While a big full-service firm such as Merrill Lynch, Pierce, Fenner & Smith might typically charge a commission of about $78 for buying 100 shares

---

stock market report

▶ *The dividend paid* by each stock, as well as the annual yield—a percentage arrived at by dividing the annual per-share dividend by the current per-share closing price.

▶ *The price-to-earnings ratio* (P/E).

▶ *The day's trading volume*—the number of shares sold—for each stock. This is an indication of investor interest in the stock and, when used in conjunction with the net gain or loss figure, of whether that interest is positive or negative. Sales will be expressed in 100s; an entry of 383, for example, would indicate the sale of 38,300 shares.

In addition, most good reports will give an indication of the market's **breadth**, the number of stocks gaining in price compared with the number losing. Breadth indices, followed regularly, can alert analysts to shifting market trends. Similarly, a listing of **most active stocks**, the 10 or 15 issues generating greatest trading volume for the day, can point to possible trends for individual issues—as well as pinpoint stocks of greatest investor interest.

of a $40 stock, major discounters like Quick & Reilly would charge approximately $41 and Discount Brokerage about $30. But watch the discounter's minimum charge. On small trades it's sometimes higher than commissions charged by full-service firms.

No broker-client relationship has to be permanent, of course. If, after a few trades, your broker has given you no reason to respect him, go elsewhere.

WHAT'S THAT BROKER SAYING?

Let's say you're ready to buy stock. You open an account with a broker. You're a radiologist, you've been impressed with all the Eastman Kodak labels on some ne-

BOX 2-2

Top stock-brokerage firms

In a poll of institutional investors, the top 10 stockbrokers were selected on the basis of research, order execution, and overall service. Only six of them (those unmarked by asterisks) accept noninstitutional —or individual—accounts:

*1. Goldman, Sachs & Co.
 2. Merrill Lynch, Pierce, Fenner & Smith Inc.
 3. Smith Barney, Harris Upham & Co. Inc.
*4. Morgan Stanley & Co. Inc.
 5. Paine Webber, Jackson & Curtis Inc.
*6. Salomon Brothers
 7. Kidder, Peabody & Co. Inc.
 8. Drexel Burnham Lambert Inc.
 9. Dean Witter Reynolds Inc.
*10. First Boston Corp.

cessities of your specialty, and you suggest to the broker that you'd like to make Kodak the first stock in what you are confident will be a growing portfolio.

"One of the Big Board's more conservative equities," the broker might say. "I think it's overdue for a split, but it's a good choice. Then shall I put in a round-lot order for EK, at the market?"

If he's a relatively inexperienced broker, he's trying to impress you; if he's an old hand, he's stupid. Nevertheless, you'll run into that kind of talk at some point, so let's decode it:

The Big Board is the nickname for the New York Stock Exchange (the American is called "the Amex," and you might even find some old-timers still calling it "The Curb"). A conservative equity, simply, is a stock not given to volatile price swings. He thinks Kodak is overdue for a "split" (it isn't, necessarily). Stocks often are split when their company's directors consider it advantageous to lower their stock's per-share price. Split a $60 share two for one, for example, and you have two $30 shares; three for one, and you have three $20 shares.

Your helpful broker would like to order a "round lot" for you. That's 100 shares or any multiple of 100 shares. Anything else would be an "odd lot." And, yes, you'll ordinarily want him to buy it "at the market." That means you'll pay whatever price "EK"—the ticker-tape symbol for Kodak—is selling for when your order reaches the stock-exchange floor. You might instead say, "No, I think we can do better than market; let's buy it at 83." To which, tapping the keys of his computer terminal, he might reply: "The last trade reported was at $84^1/_2$. You want it at 83, hold until executed or canceled." He'd then enter what's called a limit order for 100 shares of Kodak to be executed only when the stock's price fell to 83. If the price rose instead, you'd likely cancel the $83 bid and enter a higher buy order.

The stock market

"Now, ordered out or street name?" he asks. Should you tell him to "order it out," a certificate for the 100 shares, when bought, would be mailed to you by the company's transfer agent, usually a bank. But if you ordered the stock held "in street name," no certificate would change hands. Instead, the broker's firm would simply credit your account with 100 shares of Kodak held in its own portfolio.

THE NEED TO DIVERSIFY

One stock should not a portfolio make. Indeed, investment specialists will tell you that diversification among stocks is just as important as individual stock selection. That means diversifying among industries as well as among individual stock issues within an industry. It also means eventually adding such things as bonds, Treasury bills, and shares in money-market or other types of mutual funds.

How many stocks should a portfolio have? One popular answer is that no investor should hold more stocks than he can keep up with fully. An experienced, serious investor might hold 35 or 40. Another might hold no more than five. Some institutional investors—mutual funds, insurance companies, banks, etc.—hold hundreds. It's probably fair to say that 10 is a good number for the beginner, enough to assure a degree of diversification yet not too many to study thoroughly.

Even if you know at the outset what those 10 will be, you might spread the buying over a year's time, selling an issue only if a price drop made it obvious that you'd made an unwise choice. That way, you'd force yourself to study the market's swings, to become aware of the importance of timing your transactions.

Box 2-3 shows two sample portfolios, one designed for growth investors and one for those interested in income, made up of representative issues popular in today's market. There's no suggestion that you adopt them as your own—no one portfolio is right for every beginner. But a study of the statistics accompanying them will give you an understanding of what it takes to give a stock quality status.

While there are numerous forces affecting market prices, it is a stock's quality that tells over the long term. Early in 1981, for example, the Dow Jones Industrial Average (DJIA) reached an eight-year high, and investors visualized an extended bull market. By year-end 1981, however, only 909 of the 2,238 stocks then listed on the New York Stock Exchange were ahead of their 1980

text continued on page 22

BOX 2-3

Representative stock portfolios: One for growth, one for income

No one stock portfolio can meet the needs of all beginning investors. But sample portfolios such as these indicate some characteristics of high-quality stocks. Note particularly the pattern of rising earnings per share for the growth stocks. Note, too, that while income stocks yielding 10 percent and more are available, some listed here pay little more than the growth stocks listed. These are considered superior income issues for the beginner, however, because they combine relatively high dividends with potential growth in earnings that over the long term promises steadily rising income. Stocks that do pay in the 10 percent range typically are utilities, which characteristically offer little growth in either dividends or market value. These two sample portfolios were put together for MEDICAL ECONOMICS by H. Bradlee Perry, board chairman of the investment-counsel firm of David L. Babson & Co. Inc., Boston.

continued

BOX 2-3 *Representative stock portfolios* continued

	Yield (6/30/83)
GROWTH-STOCK PORTFOLIO	
Abbott Laboratories	2.1%
Air Products & Chemicals	2.1
American Express	9.1
Anheuser-Busch	2.2
Digital Equipment	0.0
Halliburton	3.9
Hewlett-Packard	0.3
Merck & Co.	3.0
Schlumberger	1.8
Wang Labs	0.2
INCOME-STOCK PORTFOLIO	
American Home Products	5.1
Dow Chemical	5.4
Exxon	8.9
General Electric	3.5
International Business Machines	3.2
Minnesota Mining & Mfg.	3.9
Mobil	6.3
Safeway Stores	5.2
Security Pacific	4.5
United Technologies	3.5

Sources: David L. Babson & Co. Inc.; Standard & Poor's Corp.

Per-share earnings ($)			Price as of 6/30/83	P/E[1]	Projected growth in dividends[2]
1981	1982	Last 12 months (to 6/30/83)			
2.01	2.37	2.47	$48^1/_8$	17	15%
4.42	3.60	3.17	$47^3/_4$	13	14
4.18	4.53	4.80	$71^1/_2$	14	12
4.79	5.67	5.84	$65^7/_8$	10	12
6.70	7.53	5.70	$119^1/_2$	23	—
4.25	5.72	3.62	$40^3/_4$	13	12
2.55	3.05	3.23	91	25	20
5.36	5.61	5.67	$92^7/_8$	15	14
4.37	4.60	4.28	54	13	15
0.68	0.88	1.08	40	34	17
3.18	3.59	3.66	$46^7/_8$	11	12
3.00	1.77	1.55	$33^1/_4$	15	9
6.44	4.82	5.08	$30^3/_8$	6	10
3.63	4.00	4.10	55	12	13
5.63	7.39	7.68	$120^1/_4$	14	14
5.74	5.37	5.40	$83^3/_4$	14	13
5.72	3.31	3.35	$31^1/_2$	9	10
2.19	3.06	3.21	$26^7/_8$	8	9
5.87	6.53	6.76	$49^1/_4$	7	11
7.71	6.73	6.95	$73^3/_8$	10	12

[1] Recent price divided by last 12 months' earnings.
[2] Projected annual growth rate of dividends for the next five years.

The stock market

price levels. The DJIA stood at 875, off 9.4 percent for the year, its worst showing since 1977.

Recession and high interest rates were taking their toll. Investors were disenchanted. And in that intemperate psychological climate, the DJIA continued its fall—to a summer-1982 low almost 100 points beneath the year-end level.

A Wall Street cliché says: "Buy when the news is bad." It's good advice—if you know *why* the news is bad and if you can honestly foresee better times ahead for a stock.

Consider Chrysler, viewed early in 1982 as a down-and-out victim of foreign competition, inept management, union pressures, high interest rates, and recession. Its common stock could be scraped off the market floor for $3 a share.

Lee Iacocca, newly arrived at the Chrysler helm, vowed—with some government concessions—to turn the company around. Iacocca succeeded in making few believers; but those who did believe were well rewarded. Chrysler common just one year later was at 25, and rising—a 733 percent gain for those who'd kept the faith when the news was bad.

Chrysler was an outstanding example. Actually, those who bought practically any stock in the summer of 1982—and held on—stood to profit. Reacting to improved economic news and lowered interest rates, the market—i.e., the DJIA—shook off its malaise. A sustained bull market was begun at a date pinpointed in hindsight as August 13, 1982.

Between January 1 and mid-May, 1983, stock prices, as measured by the DJIA, set, and broke, roughly 25 records. They'd risen more than 450 points—better than 59 percent—since the August 13 bull-market start.

And while stocks of some high-technology companies generated much of the market action, it was quality stocks, such as those making up the 30 Dow Jones industrials, that led the way with consistent gains.

Such market rises can bring on investor euphoria (a state of bliss that experienced investors view as a trap, incidentally), but the realistic investor does not easily dismiss those just-as-spectacular market drops. Change, to quote one Wall Street seer (was it Bernard Baruch?), is the stock market's only certainty. That truism is another argument for quality.

You must, in other words, recognize that each stock is an entity. That is to say that whatever "the market" is doing, whatever "they" in government are doing, and whatever "the economy" is doing, it behooves you as an investor to choose your stock purchases, and monitor them, as individual holdings.

Don't be lulled into thinking that a stock (or even a diamond) is forever. Investment counselor David L. Babson, now retired from the Boston firm bearing his name, used to advise clients: "Never buy a stock you wouldn't want to keep." But he went on to say that even stocks of endorsed quality must be regularly watched. There just might come a time when economic and financial realities put new faces on them. Then you must face up to those changes; they become stocks you wouldn't want to keep.

Investing in stocks, then, is as simple as sitting down with a broker. But making money in stocks demands a willingness to research, diversify, keep up, and remain sensitive to economic trends.

There are alternatives for the beginning investor. You'll be told of several as we move along.

Getting started in the bond market

3

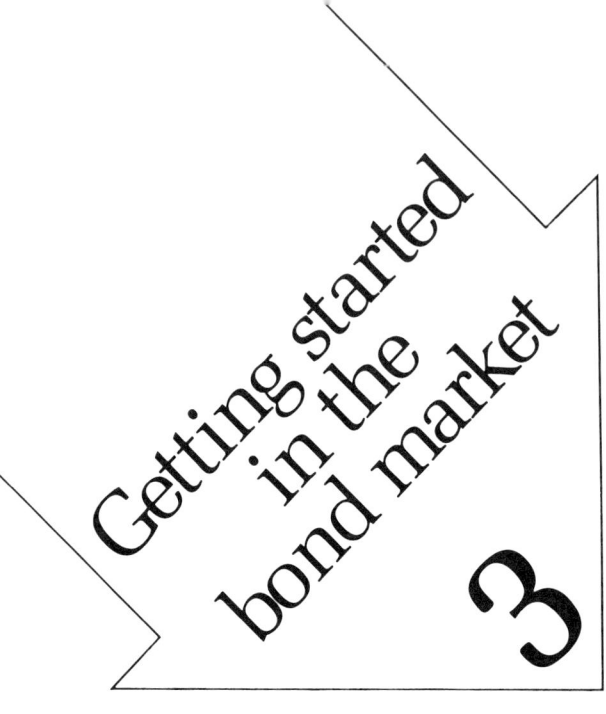

Getting started in the bond market 3

Experienced investors speak of their portfolio "mix." They know that a good investment portfolio needs more than common stocks. That might mean adding bonds, whose fixed yields tend to limit the erosion of principal in downtrending markets.

Bonds also assure full repayment of their cost, sometimes with a bonus, when held to maturity. They typically pay out interest higher than the dividend you can expect from a stock. And some of them provide substantial tax savings.

Before you can reap those rewards, you need to start at the beginning:

Think of a bond as an IOU from a corporation or some branch of government—federal, state, or local. Each bond represents an amount, usually $1,000, that the issuer has borrowed from you through an investment banker. They're "debt" issues. Stocks, by way of comparison, are "equity" issues; they represent equity—i.e., partial ownership—in a corporation.

Bonds are "senior" securities. If the issuing corporation, for example, runs into trouble and must liquidate its assets, bondholders will be among the first in line for repayment of the money they've loaned. Similarly, if hard times limit a corporation's payout to investors, bondholders will be paid their interest before holders of common stock receive their dividends; indeed, the dividends might go undeclared, meaning none will be paid.

All bonds issued today are registered. That is, they're issued to a specific investor, whose interest payments usually arrive in the mail twice a year.

There also are bearer bonds—the form once preferred for government issues—that carry no names; they're assumed to be the property of whomever has possession of them. The issue of new bearer bonds became illegal at the end of 1982, however, because the Reagan Administration feared that they contributed to income-tax cheating; since they carry no clues to ownership, more imaginative holders saw no reason to declare the income the bonds paid.

Now, the only bearer bonds around are those issued prior to 1983. The fact that most of those extant have started to trade at premium prices suggests that there's some validity to the Administration's tax-cheat theory.

Bearer bonds come complete with coupons that state the amount of interest to be paid on given dates. The bearer clips his coupons as they come due and submits them—no questions asked—to the issuer or a bank to collect his interest.

It's worth noting, too, that some bonds, especially those issued during periods of high interest rates, may be called. The issuing corporation may demand their redemption, that is, at a date of its own choosing—which usually means that it has found ways of borrowing money more cheaply. The call was once considered a very negative aspect of bonds; you bought bonds, after all, to lock up a stated rate of interest for a stated period of time.

But bond-buyer thinking has changed radically in the last few years. Bonds aren't just for holding any more. They're actively traded. Some have become what financial purists would disclaim as a contradiction of terms: "growth" bonds.

So you need to be wary of callable bonds only if your interest is in locking up an assured yield. Even then they pose no real problem. They're issued with a stated "call date" and stated call prices; the issuer guarantees that they will not be called before that stated date (this is known as "call protection"), and the call price—the price to be paid for those bonds that are called—assures buyers a fair return. More on that a bit later.

Now, let's explain away the term "growth" bond: Bond prices tend to move inversely to interest rates in general. Since a bond's own interest rate is fixed, mathematics demands that its payout—stated as a percentage of the bond's face value—must increase when the price falls—as it will do when interest rates in general are rising. Similarly, the payout percentage must fall as the market price rises. You'll see examples of that shortly.

The point here is that when interest rates in general began to soar in the late 1970s, long-term bonds issued at comparatively lower rates—4 and 5 percent, for example—suffered drastic losses in market price. It was inevitable; investors weren't about to pay $1,000 for a bond yielding $50 a year (5%) when the same money would get them a yield of $120 (12%). But if that 5 percent bond could be made to return $120, too, it would be in the running. The only way to achieve that is to bid down the price. The market makes that adjustment automatically, and the 5-percenter begins selling at discounted prices. In this case it would have to fall to roughly $415 to match the 12-percenter's payout.

Some bonds of very high quality suffered just such price drops. Foreseeing an eventual interest-rate reversal, or at least a gradual decline in interest rates, astute investors began picking up those deeply discounted bonds as growth issues. Not only were they assured yields comparable to those on high-coupon bonds, they could—by holding on—score capital gains as the bond moved toward its maturity date.

WHY INVEST IN BONDS?

Even the bluest of blue-chip stocks are subject to market swings that can be ruinous to investors. All stocks, moreover, are at the market's mercy throughout their open-ended lives. Bonds, too, can rise and fall in price, as noted above, but they promise to pay back their face value (par) at the end of their lives. That end is clearly spelled out as a maturity date.

The fixed yield that bonds offer is stated as a percentage of par, e.g., an 8 percent bond with a par value of $1,000 will pay $40 in interest every six months, or a total of $80 a year. That 8 percent yield is called the coupon rate.

But suppose rising interest rates cause the market price of that 8 percent bond to fall to 80, or $800.* The bond will continue to pay $80 annually, but its current yield—as opposed to coupon rate—will be 10 percent ($80 yield ÷ $800 price = 0.10, or 10 percent). Similarly, if the bond's price rose to 105, its current yield would drop to 7.62 percent. A bond selling below par is said to be selling at a discount, and its current yield is above the coupon rate. Above par, the bond is selling at a premium and the current yield is below the coupon rate. For the complete story on figuring bond yields, see Box 3-1.

---

*Each "point" of a bond's market price is worth $10. While a bond's face value usually is $1,000, its price is quoted as if its face value were $100. You'd pay $800 for a bond quoted at 80, for example, $1,050 for one quoted at 105, and $906.25 for one quoted at $90^5/_8$.

BOX 3-1

> ### Here's what those
>
> All bonds carry an interest rate pegged to their par value. Known as the **coupon rate**, it's simply a specified percentage of the bond's face value. A $1,000 bond with a 6 percent coupon, for example, will have a yield of $60 annually.
>
> But bond prices seldom stay at par, or face value, for long once trading in them begins. And when prices change, yields change. The figure that you're concerned with, then, is the **current yield**. Let's assume that a 6 percent bond is trading today at 92 ($920), or 8 points below par. The coupon still assures a $60 payout; so the current yield becomes 6.52 percent ($60 ÷ $920 = 0.0652, or 6.52 percent).
>
> If you're seriously interested in comparing bonds—or worried whether a fixed-income investment can keep pace with inflation—you must also consider a bond's maturity date. And you must figure **yield to maturity**. Here's a simple method of approximating that figure, sticking with that 6 percent bond, and assigning it a 1994 maturity:
>
> | | |
> |---|---:|
> | Take the face value of the bond | $1,000 |
> | and subtract the current price | −920 |
> | to get the discount from par | $80 |

The fixed features of bonds—the unchanging coupon rates and maturity dates—make them useful to investors seeking to preserve capital. Their yields, usually considerably above those of stocks, appeal to investors wanting to maximize a portfolio's income. And, as you'll see later on, some bonds provide a potential for capital gain and tax savings that endears them to tax-conscious investors.

HOW DO YOU BUY THEM?

The temptation is to answer that question with a flip "Very carefully." That would be a valid answer, but let's deal with some practicalities first.

bond-yield figures mean

Divide that discount by the years to go before maturity	$80 ÷ 10
to get the discount per year	= $ 8
and add one year's interest	+ 60
to get the total annual income	$68

Now all you need is the average of two numbers to find the yield to maturity.

The first number is total income per year divided by the current price of the bond:

$$\$68 \div \$920 = 0.0739$$

The second number is total income per year divided by the face value of the bond minus the discount per year:

$$\$68 \div (\$1{,}000 - \$8) \text{ or}$$
$$\$68 \div \$992 = 0.0685$$

Average the two and you have yield to maturity:

```
  0.0739
+ 0.0685
  0.1424 ÷ 2 = 7.12 percent yield to maturity.
```

You can buy corporate bonds from the same broker who sells you stocks. But expertise in stocks doesn't necessarily recommend him to deal in bonds. Some stockbrokers who cut their teeth on the go-go markets of the 1960s, for example, still display characteristic disdain for bonds, either because they're ignorant of the subject or not interested in the relatively low commissions bond sales bring.* Don't be overwhelmed by a broker's gener-

---

*Commissions are based on the number of bonds you buy and vary greatly with the type of brokerage firm you use. A full-service broker might charge you as much as $25 for purchasing a single bond. As the size of your order increases, the commission per bond decreases, dropping to around $5 per bond on orders of, say, 50 or more. Discount brokers charge as little as $2.50 per bond, but many impose a minimum commission that raises the cost per bond on very small orders.

osity when he offers to sell you bonds commission-free. In that event, he's selling from his own inventory, and his commission is built into the asking price. Don't hesitate to look elsewhere if your broker's knowledge or interest seems wanting.

If it's Treasury bonds you want, you might find your bank's bond department more knowledgeable. If it's municipals, especially those issued by your own city or state, you may fare better with a local brokerage house specializing in, perhaps even underwriting, such issues.

But don't go all the way with a regional house until you check its reputation with knowing bankers, accountants, and others tuned into the local financial community. A firm whose trading does not extend beyond its own state's borders doesn't always have to conform to Securities and Exchange Commission standards; there's room, therefore, for laxities that could prove expensive.

Before you can decide what type of bond and which broker you need, you'll have to decide what you want your investment to do for you. There are three main goals that bonds can accomplish.

DO YOU WANT SAFETY OF PRINCIPAL ABOVE ALL ELSE?

If so, you'll likely turn to the largest single issuer of bonds, the U.S. Government. Treasury bonds, which have a face value of at least $1,000 and mature 11 to 30 years after they're issued, are backed by the government's power of taxation and are generally considered the safest of investments. That reputation gives the Treasury a competitive edge when it goes to the public for money; so Treasury issues can—and do—pay relatively low rates of interest.

To avoid any confusion, remember that the term "Treasuries" encompasses securities other than bonds. Most notable are Treasury bills sold in a minimum denomination of $10,000 and maturing in three, six, or 12 months, and Treasury notes, sold with face values that are sometimes as low as $1,000 and maturing in a maximum of 10 years. The interest paid on all Treasuries is subject to federal income tax but is exempt from state and local taxes.

② Higher—but fully taxable—yields can be obtained from bonds offered by government agencies such as the Federal Home Loan Bank Board and the Federal National Mortgage Association. These bonds have a reputation for safety that rivals that of Treasuries; their prices, however, are more volatile.

③ You can also find safety—and the highest yields of all—in the corporate bonds issued by big business to finance operations and growth. Corporates are called mortgage bonds when they're backed by a mortgage on the firm's property and fixed assets. When secured by the general credit and potential of the issuing corporation, rather than specific assets, corporate bonds are called debentures.

Whichever form is used, you are best able to assess the soundness of a particular issue by looking at the rating it has been given by one of the independent appraisal firms, Moody's Investors Service Inc. or Standard & Poor's Corp.

Those ratings represent an assessment of the issuer's ability to pay the promised interest and, eventually, to buy back the bond at par. The top ratings, Moody's Aaa and Standard & Poor's AAA, are reserved for the likes of General Motors Acceptance Corp. and General Electric Company issues. Few specialists would advise you to go below the Moody's or Standard & Poor's A ratings if quality is your primary concern. It must be pointed out, however, that the incidence of bond defaults—Penn Central just a few years ago being a standout exception—is exceedingly low.

DO YOU WANT BONDS FOR INCOME?

Then bear in mind that the lower a bond's quality rating, the higher the interest it will likely have to pay to attract buyers. It's the old risk-and-reward theory—the more risk you take, the higher the interest you expect to be paid to take it.

Consider Indianapolis Power & Light's issue carrying a $7^1/_8$ percent interest coupon and maturing in 1998. When it was selling at $58^1/_4$ for a yield to maturity of 13.64 percent, a comparable Indiana & Michigan Electric Co. bond, with an interest coupon of only 7 percent and also maturing in 1998, was selling at $53^1/_2$ for a yield to maturity of 14.64 percent. The big difference in the two: Indianapolis P&L's rating is AA, Indiana & Michigan Electric's is BBB.

Those two utility issues exemplify another route, mentioned earlier, to maximizing income—and to achieving tax savings as well. It's buying bonds whose prices have become discounted. When those two bonds were issued, a 7 percent yield—$70 annually per bond—was ample to attract buyers at par. But a utility bond today has to yield 11 or 12 percent to stay in the running. A bond with a fixed $70 yield, then, has to drop in price in order to measure up. Thus, the Indianapolis P&L issue was bid down to $58^1/_4$, a level at which its $70 payout became a current yield of 12.02 percent ($70 divided by $582.50 = 0.12017, or 12.02%).

Let's say you bought it at $58^1/_4$, planning to hold it to maturity. You'd receive your 12.02 percent annually, and be taxed fully on it. In 1998, the bond you bought for $582.50 would reach maturity, and you'd redeem it at par, $1,000. You'd have a $417.50 gain over the $582.50—taxable at the advantageous 20 percent capital-gains rate.

Play that game with several bonds, and you have a profit worth considering.

IS IT A TAX ADVANTAGE YOU WANT?

For a purer tax advantage, look to municipal bonds—"munis" to the knowing—issued by state and local governments to finance every conceivable type of public project. Secured by revenue from the projects they serve or by the issuer's taxing power, municipals have a commendable record of safety (the 1983 debacle featuring Washington Public Power Supply System notwithstanding). Their yields are fully exempt from federal income taxes and in many cases from state and local taxes. But there's a catch: Their yields are also considerably lower than those on corporates or Treasury bonds of comparable quality.

That means you need to do some figuring to determine whether the purchase of municipals is worthwhile. Fortunately, there are comparison tables readily available to help you. Let's say you're attracted to a corporate bond, Ford Motor Co.'s $9^{1}/_{4}$s, '94—meaning a Ford bond that would yield 9.25 percent at par and that will mature in 1994. When it catches your eye, it's yielding 11 percent on its price of $83^{1}/_{4}$ ($832.50)

You know, though, that its yield is fully taxable, and you wonder if you shouldn't consider instead a tax-free municipal. Knowing that you're in the 44 percent tax bracket (a taxable income of around $50,000), you have only to consult a reference like Box 3-2 to determine which type of bond might be the better buy.

In this case, the municipal would be. The table shows that the Ford bond's taxable 11 percent is roughly equivalent in your tax bracket to a tax-free yield of 6 or $6^{1}/_{2}$ percent. And it isn't difficult these days to find municipals yielding 9 percent and better.

One caveat: Investors in municipals are not entirely certain that accurate data on issues are available. New York City's near-bankruptcy forced an improvement in financial reporting, but in this area it is far from ideal.

The bond market

Cities and states are not at present required to file anything comparable to the prospectuses that corporations must file with the SEC.

WHAT'S THE BEST WAY TO GET STARTED?
If you don't feel ready to strike out on your own, you have two alternatives in the increasingly popular bond mutual funds and bond trusts. Like mutual funds made up of stocks, bond funds comprise a number of bond issues that are professionally managed—bought and traded as managers see fit—in order to maximize investment returns. Bond trusts, on the other hand, are pools of professionally selected bonds that remain intact until they reach maturity.

Both the funds and the trusts make a lot of sense. They give you professional management at low cost and let you share the diversification in a portfolio of 50 or so bond issues with an initial investment that can be as low as $1,000.

If you're the do-it-yourself type, fine. But be careful. You'll be competing against the professionals who manage those bond funds and trusts, not to mention the ones responsible for increased activity among the big institutional investors. Bonds these days are actively traded, in search of fractional-point profits. That kind of activity has made watchfulness an imperative.

Reading the financial pages of a good newspaper regularly becomes a necessity. And if the trading idea snags your fancy, you'll want to go farther. Ask your broker for a copy of the bond reference he uses. Chances are it's Standard & Poor's *Bond Guide*, a comprehensive monthly statistical profile of all actively traded corporate bonds plus several thousand municipal bonds. It's available by subscription. Make use of the Standard & Poor's and Moody's materials in the broker's reference room.

Doing that, you'll become aware of some terms mentioned earlier, "callable," "non-callable" (often abbreviated "N/C"), and "call price." They're important terms because they bear on the life expectancy of a bond's yield.

Consider American Cyanamid's $7^3/_8$s of 2001. Cyanamid had no way of knowing, when the bond was issued

text continued on page 40

BOX 3-2

Can municipals really save you money?

Your tax bracket is the key to the answer: You need to compare taxable and tax-exempt yields at your own tax level. Here's a handy rule-of-thumb method for doing that: Subtract your tax bracket from 100 percent (let's say you're in the 44 percent bracket; then 100 minus 44 equals 56). Now divide the resulting figure into the municipal's tax-exempt yield (say the yield is 9 percent; then .09 divided by .56 equals .1607, or 16.07 percent). You'll see that the taxable investment would have to yield 16.07 percent in this example, then, to equal the municipal's tax-exempt yield of 9 percent.

There's an easier way to arrive at yield equivalents, if you can live with less precision: Just consult an equivalency table like the one on the following pages. Find your tax bracket in the table; then find the tax-exempt yield offered by the municipal you're considering. Opposite that yield, in the column beneath your tax bracket, is the approximate return you'd need to have from a taxable investment to equal the municipal's tax-exempt yield. Example: You're married, filing a joint return, with a combined taxable income of $50,000 (the 44 percent tax bracket). You're considering a municipal paying 9 percent. The table tells you, as does the rule-of-thumb example, that you'd need a taxable yield of roughly 16.1 percent to match the municipal's 9 percent.

continued

BOX 3-2 *Can municipals really save you money?* continued

	EQUIVALENT TAXABLE YIELD			
Single return (in $000s)		18.2 to 23.5		23.5 to 28.8
Joint return (in $000s)	24.6 to 29.9		29.9 to 35.2	
Tax-exempt yield	\multicolumn{4}{c}{**TAX BRACKET***}			

Tax-exempt yield	29%	31%	33%	35%
6.0%	8.5%	8.7%	9.0%	9.2%
7.0	9.9	10.1	10.4	10.8
7.5	10.6	10.9	11.2	11.5
8.0	11.3	11.6	11.9	12.3
8.5	12.0	12.3	12.7	13.1
9.0	12.7	13.0	13.4	13.8
9.5	13.4	13.8	14.2	14.6
10.0	14.1	14.5	14.9	15.4
10.5	14.8	15.2	15.7	16.2
11.0	15.5	15.9	16.4	16.9
11.5	16.2	16.7	17.2	17.7
12.0	16.9	17.4	17.9	18.5
13.0	18.3	18.8	19.4	20.0
14.0	19.7	20.3	20.9	21.5

* Applicable to tax brackets current in 1983. Source: Public Securities Association.

EQUIVALENT TAXABLE YIELD

	28.8 to 34.1		34.1 to 41.5		Over 41.5
35.2 to 45.8			45.8 to 60.0	60.0 to 85.6	Over 85.6
			TAX BRACKET*		
39%	40%		44%	49%	50%
9.8%	10.0%		10.7%	11.8%	12.0%
11.5	11.7		12.5	13.7	14.0
12.3	12.5		13.4	14.7	15.0
13.1	13.3		14.3	15.7	16.0
13.9	14.2		15.2	16.7	17.0
14.8	15.0		16.1	17.6	18.0
15.6	15.8		17.0	18.6	19.0
16.4	16.7		17.9	19.6	20.0
17.2	17.5		18.8	20.6	21.0
18.0	18.3		19.6	21.6	22.0
18.9	19.2		20.5	22.5	23.0
19.7	20.0		21.4	23.5	24.0
21.3	21.7		23.2	25.5	26.0
23.0	23.3		25.0	27.5	28.0

during 1971, whether the interest rates would climb or fall before the year 2001; therefore, the bond was made "callable," a feature that is duly noted in the various bond guides.

If interest rates rose above the bond's $7^3/_8$ percent coupon, there'd be no problem. Market action would simply discount the bond's price until the bond's yield rate reached competitive heights. But if interest rates fell significantly below the $7^3/_8$ percent coupon, Cyanamid obviously would not want to continue paying the higher rate of interest. A possible solution would be to call in the $7^3/_8$s for redemption and issue new bonds at a lower interest rate.

But what about investors who bought those bonds when they were issued and who expected to lock up an interest rate of 7.375 percent for the long term? Cyanamid took care of them when it made the bonds callable. It gave the issue an arbitrary 10 years of "call protection"—a promise, in other words, not to call in the bonds before 1981. And if it should choose to exercise the call in 1981, Cyanamid noted, it would do so at a premium—paying 104.34, or $1,043.40 for each bond.

Of course, when interest rates were near record highs during 1981, Cyanamid had no reason to call in the bonds. But, the protection ended, it still could exercise the call to satisfy sinking-fund needs before the maturity date. Should it do that, it promises, it would pay face value for the bonds called. The importance of checking a bond's call provisions, then, becomes readily apparent.

You'll also notice in the reference materials that some bonds carry a "CV" notation. They're convertibles—bonds that can be converted into the issuing corporation's common stock under specified conditions. You'll also notice that any discussion of convertibles here is conspicuously missing.

There's a reason. Convertibles, while they're useful investment instruments, are hardly for beginning investors. To use them effectively, you need a good grounding in stocks and bonds, and the interaction between the two. When you get that, you'll be ready for the advanced course.

Picking a path through the mutual-fund maze

4

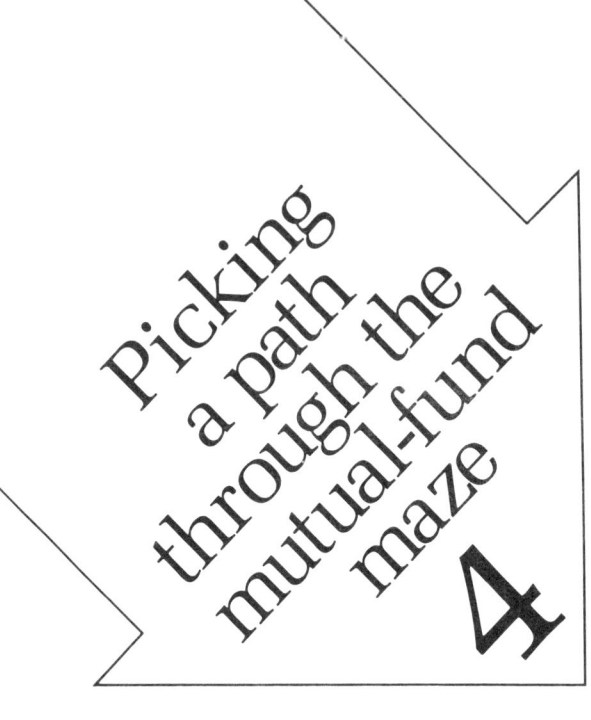

Picking a path through the mutual-fund maze
4

If you've never been offered mutual-fund shares, you're about as rare as an investor who's never sustained a loss. Fund salesmen in the last 10 years or so have become seemingly ubiquitous, and it's easy to wonder how financial publications paid their way before mutual-fund advertising came along.

The mutual-fund concept was born in Europe in the early 1900s and has been changing ever since. At its simplest, it calls for invested funds to be spread over a number of stocks and actively managed toward a desired objective, typically income or capital growth. Broadened, it allows fund managers to juggle a combination of financial instruments—common stocks, preferred stocks, bonds, convertible bonds, and cash—in an effort to achieve their aims.

And, of course, one of those aims is to attract investors whose financial input will swell the total of the fund's net assets—the amount the managers have to invest. The greater that total, the larger the management fee they collect.

The popularity of mutual funds reached its zenith in the bull market of the late 1960s. Ironically, that very popularity—which fed inordinately large sums into the funds—brought on investment excesses that led to disaster for a number of the funds and sizable losses for their shareholders. The popularity lost as a result of those so-called "go-go" excesses has been largely regained in the last five years, primarily through the high yields made possible by funds invested wholly in money-market instruments. Those high yields, of course, are a phenomenon of the high-interest-rate era. As interest rates in general decline, so will the yields. But, having been convinced again that the mutual-fund concept is valid, investors aren't likely to dismiss the funds lightly.

Previous chapters have stressed the need to reduce investment risks by diversifying—buying stocks and/or bonds that represent a variety of industries and corporations. It isn't difficult to diversify if you have a money tree that's well-leafed, but few beginning investors are so fortunate.

Therein lies a major allure of mutual funds: Investing implies risk taking. So instead of trusting one or two individual stocks with your $5,000 or $10,000 of start-up money, fund proponents ask, why not put that money into a mutual fund that spreads your risk—and your potential for gain—over 40, 50, or 100 stocks, and perhaps bonds as well?

There are other appealing qualities:

▶ Mutual funds invariably are equipped with professional managers who have the time and expertise to try to maximize the return on your investment. Able to deal in large blocks of securities, they carry market clout that you as an individual could never hope for.

▶ Funds call for relatively little money. The minimum initial investment is often as low as $100 and seldom exceeds $1,000.

▶ Up-front charges are low or frequently nonexistent as more funds take the "no-load" route and levy no sales charge. Sales charges for the so-called "load" funds usually range from 8.5 to 1.5 percent, with high-volume purchasers getting the lowest rates.

▶ Management and operating fees are fair, even if they're seldom discussed. All funds pay annual fees—typically about 1 percent of the average daily total of assets—to the companies sponsoring and promoting them. The expense reduces either income to investors or the net-asset value of fund shares, but many shareholders are never aware of it.

▶ Funds are easy to get into and out of. Brokers or independent salesmen who deal exclusively in mutual shares can put you into a load fund almost as quickly as you can uncap your check-writing pen. Getting into a no-load fund demands more initiative. The Securities and Exchange Commission requires that you make the first move by requesting a copy of the fund's prospectus. The SEC assumes that you will read the prospectus and its caveats before investing. You then submit your application and payment for shares.

Getting out is even easier. The funds must redeem their shares upon request. You simply tell the fund by phone or letter how many shares you're cashing in. The fund determines the value of your shares on the day the request is received and promptly mails you a check. A few funds levy a redemption charge—typically, 1 percent of the amount redeemed.

Probably the greatest appeal of mutual funds, though, is their diversity. Among the 750 or so mutual funds currently available, there is almost certainly one that matches your investment objective—growth, income, aggressive performance, tax savings, or whatever. Here's a sampling of the types of funds you'll encounter, and in Box 4-1 on pages 48-49 you'll find names and addresses of representative funds in each category.

Performance funds assume greater than average risks to achieve the greatest possible capital appreciation. Their portfolios often contain speculative stocks of little-known companies, albeit stocks judged by fund analysts to have exceptional growth potential. Dividends are frequently below 2 percent a year.

Growth funds strive for maximum capital appreciation consistent with safety, choosing stocks of companies with records of earnings growth and, therefore, potential to increase in market price. Growth funds typically yield annual dividends of less than 4 percent.

Growth-with-income funds attempt to balance the greater risk inherent in growth stocks with lower-risk, high-income bonds or preferred stocks. With the stock market oversensitive to interest-rate trends, these funds are a popular hedge. Dividends hover around 5 percent.

Income funds emphasize dividend-producing issues and usually include a generous lacing of bonds. Yields to shareholders generally range from about 6 percent to 10 percent or more.

Corporate-bond funds are income funds, too, with the obvious difference that they're invested almost wholly in bonds (some may hold a few preferred stocks). With interest rates still fairly high, bond funds in mid-1983 could be counted upon to provide shareholders a fully taxable return of 9 to 12 percent annually.

Municipal-bond funds shoot for maximum tax-free income from their tax-exempt bond portfolios. Mid-1983 tax-exempt yields in the 8 to 10 percent range were easy enough to come by; that's equivalent to taxable yields in the 16 to 20 percent range for investors in the 50 percent marginal tax bracket. Don't confuse municipal-bond funds with municipal-bond trusts. They're similar in that both offer a participation in tax-exempt investments. But while the funds may change the makeup of their portfolios at will—trading and selling for capital

text continued on page 50

BOX 4-1

A mutual-fund sampler

To get you started on the search for a fund that meets your investment needs, here are some representative selections, along with their telephone numbers.[1] The funds are grouped according to *United Business & Investment Report's* categories. If you don't find what you want, keep in mind there are more than 700 other funds to choose from.

For a free listing of 264 no-load funds, write to:
Investment Company Institute
1775 K Street N.W.
Washington, D.C. 20006

PERFORMANCE FUNDS
Acorn Fund
(800) 621-1660

Mathers Fund
(312) 236-8215

Over-the-Counter
Securities Fund[2]
(800) 523-2578

Putnam Voyager Fund[2]
(800) 225-1581;
(617) 423-4960
in Massachusetts

Stein Roe & Farnham
Capital Opportunities Fund
(800) 621-1142

GROWTH FUNDS
American General Enterprise[2]
(800) 231-3638

Dreyfus Fund[2]
(800) 223-5525

Fidelity Trend Fund[2]
(800) 225-6190

First Investors Fund
for Growth[2]
(212) 825-7900

Janus Fund
(800) 525-3713

Oppenheimer Directors Fund[2]
(212) 668-5100

Penn Square Mutual
(800) 523-8440

Price (Rowe) New Era Fund
(800) 638-1527

GROWTH-WITH-INCOME FUNDS
Affiliated Fund[2]
(212) 425-8720

Babson (David L.)
Investment Fund
(800) 821-5591

Colonial Fund[2]
(800) 225-2365;
(617) 426-3750
in Massachusetts

[1] 800 numbers are toll-free; check with 800 operator at (800) 555-1212 to learn whether funds listed here without 800 numbers have since added them. [2] "Load" funds, sales fee charged.

Merrill Lynch
Basic Value Fund[2]
(800) 221-7210

Pine Street Fund
(800) 221-7780

Value Line Fund[2]
(212) 687-3965

INCOME FUNDS

Hamilton Income Fund
(303) 770-2345

Putnam (George)
Fund of Boston[2]
(800) 225-1581

Shearson Income Fund[2]
(212) 321-6554

Wellesley Income Fund
(800) 523-7025

Wellington Fund
(800) 523-7025

CORPORATE-BOND FUNDS

Bond Fund of America[2]
(800) 421-0180

Fidelity Aggressive
Income Fund
(800) 225-6190

High Yield Securities[2]
(713) 654-0640 (call collect)

Keystone B-1[2]
(800) 225-1587

Northeast Investors Trust
(800) 225-6704

Price (Rowe) New
Income Fund
(800) 638-1527

MUNICIPAL-BOND FUNDS

Dreyfus Tax Exempt
Bond Fund
(800) 223-5525

Federated Tax-Free
Income Fund
(800) 245-2423

Kemper Municipal
Bond Fund[2]
(800) 621-1048

Nuveen Municipal
Bond Fund
(312) 782-2655

Price (Rowe) Tax-Free
Income Fund
(800) 638-1527

Scudder Managed
Municipal Bonds
(800) 225-2470

MONEY-MARKET FUNDS

Cash Reserve Management
(E.F. Hutton & Co.)
(212) 742-6097 (call collect)

Dreyfus Liquid Assets
(800) 223-5525

Fidelity Daily Income Trust
(800) 225-6190

InterCapital Liquid
Asset Fund
(800) 221-2685

Merrill Lynch Ready
Assets Trust
(800) 221-7210

The Reserve Fund
(800) 223-5547

gains as well as for higher yields—the trusts sell you a piece of an established tax-exempt portfolio that usually runs for a specified period. The open-ended fund concept, of course, offers bond managers greater flexibility; and, unlike the trusts, the funds are sometimes available as no-loads.

Money-market funds go all out for income from a wide variety of short-term money market instruments: bank certificates of deposit, Treasury bills and other short-term government issues, commercial paper, and bankers' acceptances—all of which you'll learn more about in the chapter that follows. Because they can buy in volume in markets that often call for minimum transactions of $1 million, money-market funds can corner highest yields. Those yields, declared daily as dividends, are spread among fund participants. Minimum investments generally range from $1,000 to $5,000. Yields vary with the ebb and flow of interest rates. They hovered in the neighborhood of 17 and 18 percent in 1981, for instance, but typically dropped below the 10 percent mark in late 1982 as interest rates in general declined and the stock market, shaking off its recession lethargy, began to attract some of the money that investors had stockpiled in the money markets.

SELECTING THE RIGHT FUND
Variations of the mutual-fund concept seem endless. Along with the thoroughly diversified funds, there are others that specialize in international stocks, foreign stocks, gold stocks, insurance-company stocks, public-utility stocks, government securities, put-and-call options, tax-exempts, new issues, and more. During the heated period of go-go investing in the late 1960s, there were even mutual funds that invested only in other mutual funds.

Before you make that first investment in a fund, you'll need to know how to select the right one. <u>Once you've determined your investment goal, you'll have to spend some time studying and comparing the funds that meet your needs.</u> You won't have any trouble finding help for this crucial step.

The funds themselves are eager to dispense information about their shares. Some brokers and salesmen know selected funds well. Wiesenberger Investment Companies Service, Lipper Analytical Services Inc., and United Business Service, among others, publish comprehensive reports comparing the investment performance of hundreds of funds—both load and no-load. The $195 yearly Wiesenberger service also provides addresses plus detailed information on each fund's management and holdings.

Your broker should be able to pull at least one of these published services from his reference shelf, even if it's a no-load fund you're checking. Failing that, he certainly can let you see a copy of Standard & Poor's *Stock Guide*, which concludes each monthly issue with a very good mutual-fund summary.

Get a prospectus from each fund that interests you and read it closely, despite its dullness. It will spell out fund weaknesses as well as strengths. A prospectus will tell you precisely what type of securities the fund deals in. It will list management fees and give a performance record that should show whether the managers are earning their keep. It will tell you whether this is an open-end fund that issues additional shares each time an investor buys in, or one of the less common closed-end funds whose shares are issued in specific quantities and traded just like those of individual stocks on major exchanges.

From the prospectus, you'll find out whether the fund offers the services you want. Does it permit switching your money into a different type of fund within the same

text continued on page 54

BOX 4-2

Some high-performing growth funds

Below are two dozen growth mutual funds, half carrying sales charges (loads) and half in the no-load category. Past records stated for them, while for the most part impressive, offer no guarantee of future performance. Such statistics are, however, clues to management capability and, as such, should be considered along with your individual investment objectives when you're choosing a fund.

The $5\frac{1}{2}$-year (12/31/77-6/30/83) tally of a $10,000 investment (which assumes reinvestment at year-end of both

NO-LOAD FUNDS	Net assets (in millions)
Constellation Growth	$ 86.9
Explorer	167.5
Founders Special	57.8
Hartwell Leverage	48.5
Janus	148.5
Keystone S-4	676.8
Loomis-Sayles Capital Development	130.7
Price (T. Rowe) New Horizons	1,373.0
20th Century Select	253.0
United Services Gold Shares	228.5
Value Line Special Situations	259.9
Weingarten Equity	83.5

dividends and capital gains) is given to indicate long-term performance over a period including both up and down markets. The 12-month and six-month figures show funds' ability to move ahead in a generally favorable market climate. Note that neither size nor load/no-load status bears directly on a fund's performance. Nor is the short-term leader necessarily a long-term leader.

Net-asset value per share (6/30/83)	6/30/83 value of $10,000 invested on 12/31/77	12-month gain, to 6/30/83	6-month gain, to 6/30/83
$26.88	$54,120	+140.0%	+55.7%
44.51	49,658	+105.5	+37.5
36.09	41,010	+107.8	+45.6
43.98	53,871	+129.5	+43.4
14.05	44,865	+ 76.4	+32.8
10.17	40,778	+156.6	+76.3
28.17	45,709	+109.5	+26.6
20.74	37,567	+ 96.0	+36.8
27.17	54,512	+106.5	+38.8
8.97	68,690	+171.0	+10.6
18.44	43,601	+ 79.4	+33.3
44.07	48,785	+114.5	+46.9

continued

BOX 4-2 *Some high-performing growth funds* continued

LOAD FUNDS	Net assets (in millions)
Fidelity Magellan	$798.0
First Investors Fund for Growth	80.7
Franklin DynaTech	22.7
Investors Research	30.3
Kemper Summit	96.0
Lord Abbett Development Growth	236.1
Massachusetts Capital Development	374.3
NEL Growth	114.5
Oppenheimer A.I.M.	278.6
Over-the-Counter Securities	59.9
Seligman Capital	101.7
Strategic Investments	96.2

Sources: Standard & Poor's Corp.; Wiesenberger Investment Companies Service.

company if your investment interests change? Is there a fee for switching? Does the fund offer a Keogh plan? A corporate retirement plan? An individual retirement account (IRA)? If it's a money-market fund, can you write checks against it? Are there any redemption restrictions? Any redemption fee?

Such considerations can be more important than whether or not you pay a sales commission—or load—up front. But there's little reason to invest in a load fund if a no-load offers the characteristics you want. That 8 percent or so charge pays salesmen, not investment managers, and reduces the amount at work for you.

Net-asset value per share (6/30/83)	6/30/83 value of $10,000 invested on 12/31/77	12-month gain, to 6/30/83	6-month gain, to 6/30/83
$38.56	$80,475	+112.4%	+43.5%
11.82	30,510	+ 98.5	+40.0
25.45	37,644	+ 98.2	+41.8
7.37	42,850	+113.0	+51.3
29.16	40,702	+ 92.4	+34.4
10.58	45,468	+100.9	+39.3
13.11	49,730	+ 87.1	+31.4
26.77	42,316	+101.3	+23.8
24.06	37,440	+ 80.1	+36.9
35.01	42,178	+ 72.5	+43.1
14.98	40,631	+135.5	+42.5
11.35	69,573	+164.0	+ 9.2

Unless you're investing in a money-market fund, make your decision with an eye to the long term. Few funds stay long at the head of any short-term performance parade. More important, it seems, is an ability to minimize losses during market downswings, to even out market peaks and troughs. Box 4-2 on pages 52-55 lists two dozen funds that have managed to do that well in the past. But past performance, as a necessary cliché goes, is no guarantee of future performance. So, when you're investing for the long term, monitor your fund's performance regularly. If it fails to measure up, consider switching.

Making the most out of the money market

5

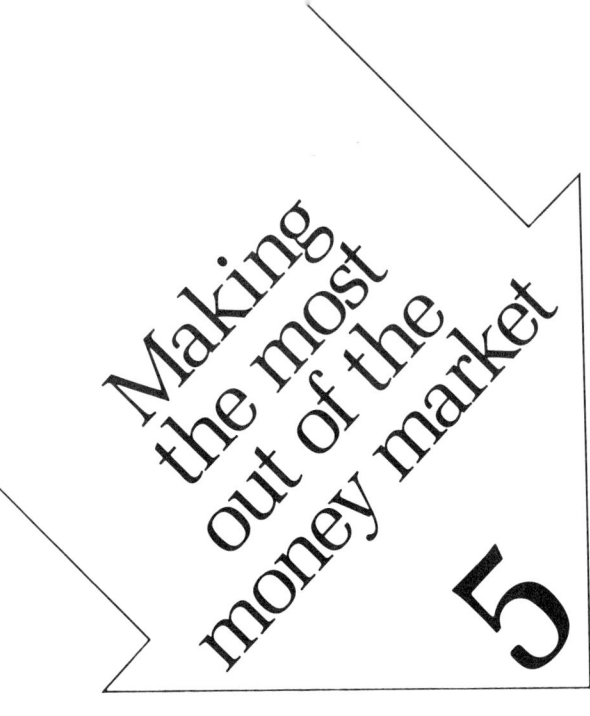

5
Making the most out of the money market

Relatively unsophisticated investors have been scoring cocktail-party points in recent years with knowing chitchat about money-market instruments. There's nothing new about these short-term, high-yield investments. Insurance companies, endowment funds, as well as other large institutional investors have used them for years.

What excited the cocktail-party circuit was growing awareness that you no longer had to plunk down at least $100,000 if you wanted the advantages of money-market instruments for yourself. These days, banks and savings institutions offer some of these instruments for as little as $10,000, while money-market mutual funds have reduced the ante to $1,000 or even less.

It's only fair to note at the outset, however, that money-market enthusiasm rises and falls in practically the same tempo as interest rates. It was interest rates climbing to double-digit levels, in fact, that spurred formation of most of the money-market mutuals.

You can be sure that in periods of lower interest rates—periods that typically give rise to bullishness in the stock market—cash will come out of the money-market instruments and go into stocks; investors, after all, go where the promise of growth seems greatest. But there always will be a place for money-market investments.

Just what do money-market instruments offer? Traditionally, their greatest attraction has been liquidity. Investors who want their money back—perhaps to take advantage of a long-term opportunity—have no trouble selling the instruments on an active secondary market. In fact, the process is so easy that the instruments are often referred to as "cash equivalents."

Equally important, however, are the attractive rates of return the instruments offer—always a notch above the competition. Add a high degree of safety to those benefits and you have good reason for learning what money-market instruments are all about, whether you're an individual looking for a small investment or a member of an incorporated practice whose retirement fund can swing the money demanded by most of the instruments in their pure form. We'll start with a quick rundown of the various instruments.

MONEY-MARKET INSTRUMENTS FOR THE BIG BOYS

With a few exceptions that your bank or broker can tell you about, these call for a minimum investment of $100,000, well beyond the means of most beginning investors. You can, however, get a piece of this action by buying shares in a money-market mutual fund. The idea is to make the most out of day-to-day shifts in yields in such instruments as these:

▶ Bankers' acceptances. You might call these a bank's way of laying off its bets. The bank agrees to accept the debt of a company—that is, to lend it money—by providing a line of credit. To assure the necessary flow of cash, the bank sells portions of that acceptance to investors. The bank—not the company—is ultimately responsible for paying back the investors' capital. Bankers' acceptances carry very short maturities, none longer than nine months.

▶ Certificates of deposit. They're simply a means of lending money to a bank or savings and loan association. Most of us know the CD as a six-month or one-year certificate that offers an interest rate higher than passbook savings; we'll see some running for five years, or more—and they're in rather small denominations. In the world of higher finance, however, CDs are in the $100,000 class. Their maturities are calculated in days—usually no fewer than 30 days and no more than 365, although a wider variety of maturities are developing with the growth in popularity of money-market investments.

▶ Commercial paper. If your son asks you to advance him $1 to stock his lemonade stand and gives you an IOU promising to repay $1.10, you're dealing in commercial paper. Commercial paper is nothing more than negotiable promissory notes issued by big corporations. The notes usually are payable within 30 or 60 days, never more than 270 days.

INSTRUMENTS FOR THE LITTLE GUY

Bankers' acceptances, CDs, and commercial paper have obvious appeal for big-time investors. Individuals can get similar yields and comparable safety with modest outlays for such instruments as these:

▶ Treasury bills. Auctioned by the government every Monday (or the preceding Friday when Monday is a holiday), Treasury bills are issued in denominations as low as $10,000. Maturities are three, six, or 12 months. (Don't confuse T-bills with longer-term Treasury notes and bonds.) The bills can be sold through a bank or broker if you need to have your money before they reach maturity.

It isn't hard for you to take part in the weekly T-bill auction. Any Federal Reserve bank (see Box 5-1, pages 62-63) can supply you with a noncompetitive tender form. Mail the form, along with a bank teller's check or certified personal check, in time for it to arrive at the Federal Reserve bank in your district by 1:30 p.m. Eastern time on the day of the auction. Because your tender is noncompetitive, you'll pay the average price of all the bids that the Treasury accepts. The Treasury will immediately mail you your interest—the difference between the price and the bill's face value.

Let's say the average price of a 26-week maturity T-bill with a face value of $10,000 was $9,512.40. To figure your annual rate of return—called the coupon yield—divide that price into the $487.60 in interest you'll receive. Double the result to adjust for a full year, and you come up with an annual yield of 10.25 percent.

Their payoff comes in the form of a discount right up front. Suppose you put $9,512.40 into a $10,000 six-month bill. Within a week, you'll receive Uncle Sam's check for half a year's interest. You can then invest the interest in something else, without waiting out the bill's 26-week term.

The income is exempt from state and local income taxes. That's no minor consideration in some states. Take New York State, for example, where the top bracket is 14 percent. If you bought a T-bill there, the annual 8 percent return, after having been boosted to 10.25 percent because of the discount in the example above, would effectively be pushed up by nearly another point. In other words, a New York investor would have to earn about 11.25 percent on a bank CD to equal the after-tax yield on an 8 percent T-bill.

There's no early-withdrawal penalty. If an emergency forces you to cash in a CD, you forfeit at least three months' interest. In contrast, T-bills can be sold on the secondary market through a bank or a stockbroker. There's usually a sales fee of $30 or so, but that's only a fraction of what you'd lose if you were forced to redeem a CD early.

BOX 5-1

Where Uncle Sam sells T-bills

The Federal Reserve has banks in the 13 cities listed, and there are 37 other Federal Reserve offices around the country. You may buy Treasury bills in person at any of those offices. You may also purchase them by mail by writing to the Federal Reserve bank nearest you or the Bureau of the Public Debt in Washington. There will be instructions with the forms, but

Federal Reserve Bank	
Atlanta	104 Marietta St., N.W. Atlanta, Ga. 30303
Boston	600 Atlantic Ave. Boston, Mass. 02106
Chicago	230 S. LaSalle St., Box 834 Chicago, Ill. 60690
Cleveland	1455 E. Sixth St., Box 6387 Cleveland, Ohio 44101
Dallas	400 S. Akard St., Station K Dallas, Tex. 75222
Kansas City	925 Grand Ave., Federal Reserve Station, Kansas City, Mo. 64198
Minneapolis	250 Marquette Ave. Minneapolis, Minn. 55480

▶ Money-market certificates. You might know these as thrift certificates, savings certificates, or even six-month CDs. They're the $10,000 short-term certificates through which banks borrow money from you.

Maturing in 26 weeks, they offer yields pegged to 26-week Treasury bills. Note that the Treasury announces its T-bill rates on Monday afternoons, while banks an-

you should also request the free booklet, "Basic Information on Treasury Notes and Bills." Since there is a choice of three different maturities, specify which tender form you want.

A bank or brokerage house will do this for you for about $30, but why cut into your profits when it's so easy to do it yourself?

Federal Reserve Bank	
New York	33 Liberty St., Federal Reserve P.O. Station New York, N.Y. 10045
Philadelphia	100 N. Sixth St., Box 66 Philadelphia, Pa. 19105
Richmond	701 E. Byrd Ave., Box 27622 Richmond, Va. 23261
St. Louis	411 Locust St., Box 442 St. Louis, Mo. 63166
San Francisco	400 Sansome St., Box 7702 San Francisco, Calif. 94120
Washington, D.C.	Bureau of the Public Debt Securities Transaction Branch Washington, D.C. 20226

nounce their certificate yields on Thursdays. If you're alert to the Tuesday morning financial pages, you know in advance what the certificates' yields will be two days hence. You can make use of that 48-hour period to buy a current CD if yields are about to drop, to delay your purchase if yields will rise, or to seek out another investment altogether.

Unfortunately, these money-market certificates have a major drawback: There's no market for their resale. You must redeem them with the institution that issued them,

BOX 5-2

Representative minimum initial

Capital Preservation Fund 459 Hamilton Ave., Palo Alto, Calif. 94301	$ 1,000
Cash Reserve Management Trust (E.F. Hutton) 1 Battery Park Plaza, New York, N.Y. 10004	10,000
Daily Cash Accumulation Fund P.O. Box 300, Denver, Colo. 80201	2,500
Dreyfus Liquid Assets 600 Madison Ave., New York, N.Y. 10022	2,500
Fidelity Daily Income Trust 82 Devonshire St., Boston, Mass. 02109	10,000
First Variable Rate Fund for Government Income 1700 Pennsylvania Ave., N.W. Washington, D.C. 20006	1,000
InterCapital Liquid Assets Fund (Dean Witter Reynolds) 130 Liberty St. New York, N.Y. 10006	5,000
Kemper Money Market Fund 120 S. LaSalle St., Chicago, Ill. 60603	1,000

Source: Donoghue's Money Fund Directory of Holliston, Mass.

and you're penalized if you do so before they reach maturity. In that case your yield then becomes less than your money would have earned in a passbook savings account.

The certificates also tend to be most popular when interest rates reach new highs and seem vulnerable to a setback. Yet it can be argued that that's precisely the time when you should be investing in long-term bonds, nailing down high yields for years instead of only 26 weeks.

text continued on page 68

investments in money-market funds

Liquid Capital Income Fund 731 National City Bank Building Cleveland, Ohio 44114	$1,000
Merrill Lynch Ready Assets Trust 165 Broadway, New York, N.Y. 10006	5,000
Money Mart Assets 100 Gold St., New York, N.Y. 10038	1,000
National Liquid Reserves 605 Third Ave., New York, N.Y. 10158	2,500
Paine Webber Cash Fund 815 Connecticut Ave. N.W. Washington, D.C. 20006	5,000
The Reserve Fund 810 Seventh Ave., New York, N.Y. 10019	1,000
Rowe Price Prime Reserve Fund 100 E. Pratt St., Baltimore, Md. 21202	2,000
Scudder Managed Reserves 175 Federal St., Boston, Mass. 02110	1,000

BOX 5-3

Other parking slots for idle cash

Instrument	Recent yield	Original maturity	Relative safety	Minimum investment
Savings accounts				
Ordinary passbook	5.50%	No restriction	Both highest (insured to $100,000)	None
Passbook time deposits	6.00	90 days		$100
Certificates of deposit		(Other CDs mature in as long as 8 years)	Highest (insured to $100,000)	Typically $1,000-$2,500
18 months	10.55			
6 months	9.56			
3 months	9.13			
Treasury bills		3-12 months	Highest (backed by U.S. Government)	$10,000
3 months	9.13			
6 months	9.31			
12 months	9.36			
U.S. agency short-term notes	10.86	Typically 3 months or longer	Very high	$5,000-$10,000; some higher
Municipal short-term notes (tax-exempt)	5.80*	1 month to 1 year	Fairly high	$5,000; usually traded in 25,000 lots

*Six months.

The beginning investor

How or where to buy	Special features
Mutual savings banks or savings and loan associations; also commercial banks at lower interest rates	Day-to-day accounts generally earn more interest than grace-day accounts, but latter type pays interest from first of month on funds deposited by 10th day
Mutual savings banks or savings and loan associations; also commercial banks at lower interest rates	Interest compounded periodically and payable at maturity, but taxable annually; rate is guaranteed for full term, but lower rate (plus penalty) will be applied on premature withdrawal
Commercial banks or brokers; or directly from Federal Reserve (no fee)	Backed by "full faith and credit" of U.S. Government; interest is earned on discount basis—difference between purchase price and face value or resale amount is interest income (reportable on federal return for year realized); interest is exempt from state and local taxes
Commercial banks or brokers; some new issues can be purchased from Federal Reserve or underwriters without commission	Issued by federal agencies or by agencies under federal sponsorship (sponsored-agency obligations are not directly guaranteed by U.S. Government); interest is usually exempt from state and local income taxes; notes can generally be resold before maturity
Commercial banks or brokers	Safest notes are those rated MIG-1 or MIG-2 by Moody's; interest is exempt from tax by U.S. and issuer's state; ease of resale before maturity depends on financial condition of issuer and size of issue

continued

BOX 5-3   *Other parking slots for idle cash*   continued

Instrument	Recent yield	Original maturity	Relative safety	Minimum investment
Bankers' acceptances	9.70*	1 to 6 months	High	$5,000; often higher
Commercial paper	9.45*	1 to 9 months	Variable	$25,000

*Six months. Sources: Federal Reserve Bank, *Barron's*, *The Wall Street Journal*, Salomon Brothers.

WHAT'S AN INDIVIDUAL TO DO?

That question brings us full circle to money-market mutual funds. They're the best game in town for the income seeker who wants to take advantage of the high yields and safety of money-market instruments.

As Chapter 4 pointed out, you need no more than $1,000—and sometimes even less—to get into these funds (see Box 5-2, pages 64-65). Most allow subsequent investments of $100 or $500. You can get out at any time without penalty. You can, in fact, write checks against your account—usually for a minimum amount of $500—if you need cash.

Not all funds achieve the same results, of course. Measure those yields against what's being paid on pure money-market instruments to determine just how well the

How or where to buy	Special features
Commercial banks or brokers	These trade obligations guaranteed by banks are suitable mainly for institutional investors but are sometimes available to individuals at attractive yields (discount basis); can usually be resold before maturity
Commercial banks or directly (without fee) from underwriter dealers and some issuers (e.g., General Motors Acceptance Corp.)	Issued on discount basis by major private corporations, sometimes with bank backing; only top-rated (A-1 or Prime-1) paper should be considered for individual investment; resale may be restricted to specific dealers

various funds stack up. Current money-market yields are published daily in *The Wall Street Journal* and in many of the larger newspapers under "Money Rates."

Two notes of caution: While most funds charge no sales fee, all have operating expenses that are passed on to shareholders. Current yields quoted by a few funds ignore that expense, which means their reported yields are inflated. Others are figured as net yields, adjusted for operating expenses. You should expect a good fund to achieve yields, after adjustment for expenses, of 0.25 to 0.75 of a percentage point above the prevailing rate on 26-week Treasury bills.

Secondly, the funds *do* follow prevailing interest rates. While that makes their yields extraordinarily attractive when interest rates are rising, it also means that such funds are not a good long-term investment. When interest rates start to fall, returns from money-market mutual funds are likely to drop sharply—a signal to bail out and lock in the best possible long-term yields from other forms of investment.

But couple the current yields with the cocktail-party points your new knowledge will bring, and you too can enjoy a big return on money-market instruments.

OTHER WAYS TO EARN MONEY WITH SPENDING MONEY

Money-market funds, Treasury bills, and six-month CDs are just three of the short-term investments you should consider. Several others can provide high yields for individuals who have $5,000, $10,000, or even $25,000 to invest. Their interest rates fluctuate in fairly close relationship to one another, but they're often a little higher than those of long-term investments. One or another of these parking places should give you earnings that will offset—or even exceed—increases in the cost of living. The yields shown in Box 5-3, pages 66-69, are for midyear 1983. Where applicable, discount rates have been converted to the equivalent interest basis.

Tiptoeing profitably into real estate

6

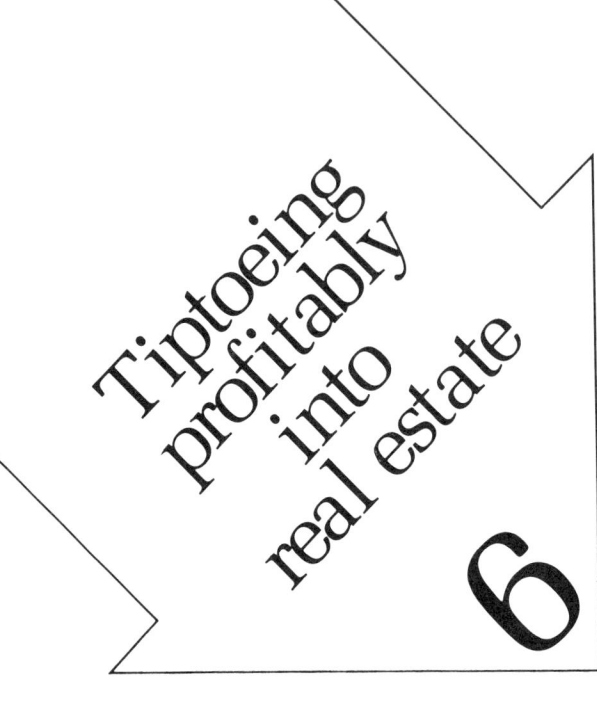

Tiptoeing profitably into real estate

6

Chances are, you're a real-estate investor already. You are if you've acquired your own home or invested in your own office building.

Some of what we say here will apply to those important investments, the first that any physician should make. For the most part, though, we'll assume that you want to take a broader look at real-estate investing, either to learn what's out there or to refresh your memory of the territory. The intent is to provide enough information to help you decide whether real-estate investing is for you.

As Box 6-1 illustrates, real estate is an extremely popular form of investment, especially among doctors. Undeveloped land and rental housing are favored by physicians of all ages, but farm acreage rates high mainly with your older colleagues. Commercial property's appeal is strongest for doctors in midcareer, who can generally best afford the risks that go along with the large potential rewards.

BOX 6-1

Which realty investments doctors favor

Age group	Type of investment	Percentage of M.D.s who hold it	Median equity*
30-39	Farm acreage	5%	$23,000
	Raw land (nonfarm)	17	17,000
	Rental housing	14	34,000
	Commercial property	9	38,000
40-49	Farm acreage	11	63,000
	Raw land (nonfarm)	21	30,000
	Rental housing	26	52,000
	Commercial property	20	55,000
50-59	Farm acreage	15	75,000
	Raw land (nonfarm)	26	29,000
	Rental housing	22	63,000
	Commercial property	19	65,000
60-69	Farm acreage	18	75,000
	Raw land (nonfarm)	25	56,000
	Rental housing	18	58,000
	Commercial property	12	53,000
All M.D.s	Farm acreage	12	67,000
	Raw land (nonfarm)	22	29,000
	Rental housing	21	52,000
	Commercial property	16	57,000

*Among those having any. All figures in this table apply to office-based M.D.s.
Source: MEDICAL ECONOMICS Financial Survey, 1980.

WHY GET INTO REAL ESTATE AT ALL?

An easy answer is that man is naturally an acquisitive animal, and there's no more basic acquisition than land. Perhaps more important, real-estate investments—properly chosen and managed—promise excellent profits that are most often treated kindly by the Internal Revenue Service.

Consider some reasons:

▶ Profits from properties held longer than one year are usually taxed at favorable capital-gains rates.

▶ Interest paid on mortgage loans is tax-deductible.

▶ The IRS accepts the fact that no building lasts forever. That means investors can take annual deductions for depreciation—paper losses that will reduce income tax—even though the building's market value may actually be increasing every year.

▶ Real estate held as an investment may be exchanged for "like kind" property to delay payment of any tax on profits. "Like kind" is broadly interpreted: An office building, for example, could be exchanged for a warehouse of equal value, because both properties are commercial. (But if you received cash as well as the warehouse for your office building, the cash payment would represent a taxable gain.)

STARTING OUT IN REAL ESTATE

With taxes such a vital consideration, you'd do well to begin with some serious reading on the subject. You'll find any number of pertinent publications in the business-reference section of public libraries. Look for publications copyrighted in 1982 or later. Earlier books won't reflect the sweeping tax changes enacted since then.

To be sure of your tax information, study the latest issues of IRS publications. Or, in the interest of lucidity, check the interpreted versions—such as *U.S. Master Tax*

Guide, published by Commerce Clearing House Inc., and J.K. Lasser's *Your Income Tax*.

Having dipped into one aspect of real estate—taxes—you have a number of others to consider. These include the degree of risk, liquidity (can you sell without significant loss if you need money?), rate of return, and the amount of time and effort your property will demand from you.

Before you're overwhelmed by all of this, take a tip from knowledgeable real-estate investors: Assemble a team of assistants. At the very minimum, you'll need help from a real-estate broker you trust, and possibly from an appraiser. If you're eyeing a complex deal, try to get the help of a CCIM—a certified commercial-investment member of the Realtors National Marketing Institute—with expertise in investment real estate. Be prepared, too, to call in your accountant and a tax-savvy attorney.

HOW IT ALL WORKS

Let's run through an example of a simplified real-estate investment just to see how profits—or losses—are created. Note the influential weight of tax rules.

Suppose you can muster $35,000 to invest and can spare $650 monthly from practice income toward the investment. Excellent, the real-estate broker says; that's more than ample to swing a $125,000 fourplex. With your good credit rating, you can borrow about $90,000 from a bank. Or perhaps the building's present owner, aware that money is tight and anxious to close the deal, will agree to a purchase-money mortgage. That arrangement, in which the seller becomes the lender, usually will allow you to negotiate an interest rate lower than the prevailing bank rate.

You check out the 5-year-old building and find it to be in good repair. It's well located in a white-collar residential neighborhood just east of the city center. You and your accountant can find no financial red flags in the owner's books. Each of the four apartments is rented for $375 a month, and—despite inflation—rents were last raised two years ago.

You agree to buy, using your $35,000 as a down payment and accepting the seller's offer of a 10-year purchase-money mortgage at 15 percent interest.

You'll put that $650 a month from practice income into a liquid, interest-bearing account to provide a minimum of $7,800 a year. This will cover insurance, taxes, and maintenance.

Now that you're a landlord, your first move will be to raise those low rents—to $450 a month per unit. That'll bring in $21,600 a year, assuming that you maintain 100 percent occupancy.

But wait, you say. Who wants to be a landlord for the rest of his life? No problem. As an investor, you can and should set goals to suit your personal situation. Let's say you count on selling the property after one year, even though most real-estate investments would be held longer. An appraiser tells you that you can reasonably expect a price of $150,000, considering inflation and continued strong demand for housing. Where would that put you as an investor?

The apartments brought you $21,600 in income during the year. Subtract from that $12,150 in interest payments and $7,800 for taxes, insurance, maintenance, and other expenses. That leaves you with a net income of $1,650 in cash from the apartments, but real estate also provides an important bookkeeping deduction for depreciation.

Using rules outlined later in this chapter, you could deduct $8,333 for depreciation of your building under the straight-line method. That write-off would wipe out any taxes on the rental income and leave you with a $6,683 loss on your books. Deduct that loss against practice income, and in the 50 percent bracket you'd save more than $3,300 in taxes; in the 42 percent bracket, a little more than $2,800.

The combination of rents and tax deductions gives you $4,991 in income. Balance that against the $9,000 you've shelled out in monthly payments on the principal of your mortgage, and you're left with an operating loss—real-estate savants call it a negative cash flow—of $4,009 for the year. In this case, that's not a bad deal. You'll still come out ahead.

Suppose you sell for the $150,000 the appraiser projected. Figure on paying 6 percent of that—$9,000—to the broker who handles the sale, leaving you with a long-term capital gain of $20,000. Since long-term capital gains are taxed at a lower rate than ordinary income, you'd pay $4,000. Subtracting that tax would leave you with a gain of $16,000—a profit of 36 percent on the $44,000 you'd invested through the down payment and amortization.

One reason you'd rack up a score that large would be that you made your initial $35,000 do the work of $125,000. That's called leverage—borrowing money to increase the clout of the funds you're able to invest. But any mention of leverage demands a caveat: While it can magnify gains excitingly, leverage can magnify losses, too, and is not to be toyed with without professional help. That's one more reason any serious entry into the real-estate investment field should be made with professional handholding.

Not all real-estate deals will be as lucrative as this example, but many will make the example look like a penny-ante game. The point is that all successful real-estate investments are built on the idea of using tax measures and leverage to greatest advantage.

If you're convinced that with expert help you can handle the challenge of real estate, your next step is to figure out how deeply you wish to be involved. You must decide, too, whether you want to be an active or passive real-estate investor.

"ACTIVE" INVESTMENTS FOR GREATEST DIVERSITY

Active investments include sale-and-leasebacks, triple-net leases, and a variety of other ways in which commercial or residential properties are used to generate cash flow and/or tax benefits.

▶ A sale-and-leaseback is a sophisticated means of playing to real estate's tax advantages. It's so sophisticated, in fact, that no beginning investor should get involved without the help of an expert.

Here's how a sale-and-leaseback works: A fast-food chain—we'll call it Mama's—buys a corner lot in your town that it considers an ideal location for a Mama's restaurant. But Mama's wants no part of the real-estate business, and it puts out the word to the real-estate and financial communities that it's in the market for a leaseback. Your financial adviser suggests that you take on the restaurant as a tax shelter.

In a typical deal, Mama's will sell the lot to you at a price, if you'll construct a restaurant precisely to Mama's specifications. With Mama's plans in hand, you negotiate a long-term loan to finance the building's construction. Or Mama's might even construct the building and sell it to you along with the lot.

When the building is completed, you lease the property back to Mama's. Mama's gets a hand-picked location with a long-term lease and the ability to write off leasing costs as a business expense. You get enough guaranteed income to amortize your mortgage loan; yet that income is likely to become a loss for tax purposes after you've deducted depreciation, loan interest, maintenance, and other costs. You'd use that loss, of course, to offset taxable practice income. And if you chose to sell the property eventually, your gain would be taxed at the advantageous capital-gains rate.

▶ A triple-net lease would go well as an extension of the Mama's deal. You'd accept Mama's leaseback offer but specify that payments to you would be net after property taxes, insurance, and maintenance. In other words, Mama's would relieve you of responsibility for that trio of necessities. They're easy write-offs against Mama's income, but they have no value to your tax-shelter program. You might simplify matters further by insisting at the outset upon an "escalation" clause or a "percentage" override. The first would grant you an automatic rent increase each time the inflation rate rose. The latter would give you a percentage of Mama's gross once the gross exceeded a specified level.

Active real-estate investments aren't always suitable for physicians; they simply require too much looking after. A frequent solution is to line up professional management for the apartment house, shopping center, office building, or whatever. The cost can be deducted as a business expense, heightening your property's attributes as a tax shelter.

"PASSIVE" INVESTMENTS FOR MINIMAL BOTHER

Limited partnerships and real-estate investment trusts are the most prominent ways to get into the real-estate market if you're not ready to take an active role.

▶ Limited partnerships have become a popular route to passive investments. Headed by general partners who choose and manage the investment property, they allow small investors—the limited partners—to share in the fortunes of large developments, often for as little as $5,000.

Partnership participations may be offered by real-estate brokers interested in obtaining financing for a commercial project. Often organized by contractors, a wide variety of partnership offerings have been made available in the last five years or so through major stock brokerage firms.

Limited partnerships preserve many of the tax advantages of active investment in real estate, but they have a major drawback: As a limited partner, you have no voice in how the investment is managed. That's why it's crucial to examine the general partners' performance record, which you'll find in the partnership prospectus. Chapters 8 and 9 explore limited partnerships and real-estate tax shelters in more detail.

▶ **Real-estate investment trusts (REITs)** provide a direct play in real estate through the stock market, but offer no special tax advantages. Just as mutual funds buy stocks and bonds, equity REITs use pooled funds to deal in actual properties, while mortgage REITs invest in portfolios of mortgages. Shares of both kinds of REITs are listed on the stock exchanges or traded in the over-the-counter market.

Some REITs have had a troubled past, primarily because they were caught with nobody to sell their properties to when the boom-time bubble burst in the mid-1970s. REIT shares generally have fared well since, though, and their advocates insist that the industry has attained a responsible maturity. Certainly it is more cohesive now than it was in the past. Through the National Association of Real Estate Investment Trusts (NAREIT), it now readily discloses a wealth of information about itself.

You may obtain a list of REITs by writing to the association at 1101 17th Street N.W., Washington, D.C. 20036. If that whets your appetite for more information, ask for a copy of *REITs Quarterly*, a comprehensive research report covering the industry.

WHY NOT RAW LAND?

You'll notice that we haven't mentioned undeveloped land. Not that raw land can't be an excellent investment; it can be among the best. Certainly it's the most popular among your fellow doctors, as Box 6-1 shows. But for the beginning investor—for any investor—it has to be called a speculation, not an investment.

Location is all-important. Is the land in the path of profitable development? Who knows? Many an expected real-estate fortune has dissolved into nothing with a government decision to reroute a major highway.

The key, say some of those who've been successful, is to foresee a use for a tract and then convince developers of the potential for profit. It's also essential that you buy the land cheaply. You'll be stuck with taxes and financing costs for as long as you hold it, and you don't know how long that might be.

Even if you never work up to the sophistication of investing in raw land, however, you can't afford not to be aware of the potential in real estate. Whether it's your home, your office, or an outside venture, a well-planned real-estate investment can provide your most secure base for dealing with a turbulent economy.

DEPRECIATION MADE COMPARATIVELY SIMPLE

Real-estate investments can be both rewarding and complex. Internal Revenue Service rules governing depreciation are factors in both characteristics.

Depreciation is basically a bookkeeping transaction. Originally, it hinged on the idea that every building or piece of equipment has a "useful life." As each year of that life passes, the owner is allowed to deduct from current income a portion of what he originally invested—even if the property is growing in value.

How do you determine that useful life? You can use either Treasury Department guidelines or experience with similar buildings. A beginner will definitely need the help of a good tax accountant, both for that question and for the other complexities of depreciation. An expert can also guide you safely through the rule changes of recent years. For the time being, however, here are some streamlined examples of how depreciation works. Note that all values in these examples apply only to buildings. The land under them cannot be depreciated, and its value doesn't enter into our calculations.

▶ Straight-line depreciation is by far the simplest method and can be applied to all kinds of real estate. It assumes that a property will depreciate equally each year over selected depreciation periods that may be 15, 35, or 45 years. Suppose, for instance, that you buy a small office building for $100,000, hoping to profit from its rental income while depreciating it over 15 years (the 1981 tax-law amendments say most property placed in service after 1980 must be depreciated over 15 years). You'd simply divide the building's cost by 15 to determine the depreciation allowable each year. You'd get an annual deduction of $6,666.67, or 6.67 percent, from your income.

If you sold the building before a year elapsed, however, you'd have to pay ordinary income tax on the proceeds and would not be allowed the depreciation deduction. That's called recapture. If you held the property longer than a year, not only would you be protected from recapture of any straight-line depreciation, you'd also qualify for favorable long-term capital-gains tax rates on any profit when you eventually sold. Tax considerations get trickier when you move on to more complicated methods of depreciation.

▶ Declining-balance depreciation, known as the accelerated cost recovery system (ACRS), speeds up the rate at which you can claim deductions. This system doesn't increase the total of deductions to which you're entitled, but it allows you to write off more of your investment in your initial period of ownership before 1985. In 1985, ACRS depreciation must be switched to the straight-line method.

For most types of real property bought or constructed after 1980, the Treasury provides a 15-year depreciation period and dictates an accelerated cost recovery system (ACRS) to cover it. The system incorporates new tax rules calling for use of the 175 percent declining-balance method of depreciation and a mandatory switch to straight-line depreciation after 1985.

The system, typical of Treasury efforts to "simplify," actually muddies the depreciation waters. It does not, for example, apply to residential rental properties; they may be depreciated by the 200 percent declining-balance method. So it may be comforting to know that straight-line depreciation can always be used. Along with its simplicity, straight-line depreciation offers another advantage: There's no recapture of depreciation required when the property is sold and a capital gain is realized. Conversely, when there's a capital gain on the sale of property depreciated under an accelerated method, the depreciation is subject to recapture.

To see how all this works, consider the same $100,000 office building as before and assume it was purchased in January. Now, take a look at the Treasury's depreciation schedule set out in Box 6-2, on page 84. You'll see that the month in which the property was put into service determines the depreciation rate.

Your depreciation in the first year would be at a 12 percent rate, or $12,000. The rate would decline in the second year to 10 percent, or $10,000; in the tenth to 5 percent ($5,000), etc., until the full $100,000 value was recovered.

Real estate   83

BOX 6-2

ACRS depreciation rates, nonresidential property

To determine the applicable percentage of depreciation, use the column representing the month in the first year the property was placed into service.

Recovery year	Month property was placed into service											
	1st	2nd	3rd	4th	5th	6th	7th	8th	9th	10th	11th	12th
1	12%	11%	10%	9%	8%	7%	6%	5%	4%	3%	2%	1%
2	10	10	11	11	11	11	11	11	11	11	11	12
3	9	9	9	9	10	10	10	10	10	10	10	10
4	8	8	8	8	8	8	9	9	9	9	9	9
5	7	7	7	7	7	7	8	8	8	8	8	8
6	6	6	6	6	7	7	7	7	7	7	7	7
7	6	6	6	6	6	6	6	6	6	6	6	6
8	6	6	6	6	6	6	5	6	6	6	6	6
9	6	6	6	6	5	6	5	5	5	6	6	6
10	5	6	5	6	5	5	5	5	5	5	6	5
11	5	5	5	5	5	5	5	5	5	5	5	5
12	5	5	5	5	5	5	5	5	5	5	5	5
13	5	5	5	5	5	5	5	5	5	5	5	5
14	5	5	5	5	5	5	5	5	5	5	5	5
15	5	5	5	5	5	5	5	5	5	5	5	5
16	—	—	1	1	2	2	3	3	4	4	4	5

Had you chosen to use straight-line depreciation, your deduction each year would have been the same—$6,667 ($100,000 divided by 15 years = $6,667, or 6.666 percent, per year). Considering that your deductions under the accelerated method would be taxed as ordinary income upon sale of the property, the straight-line method becomes preferable—except for those who need the large up-front deductions to offset other income in the early years of the investment.

This seems a good time to point up a statement made earlier: Real-estate investing is made dangerously complex by tax laws and the extent to which taxes affect its bottom line. You've seen how depreciation can maximize gains on commercial property—if it's straight-line. And you've seen how depreciation-recapture rules can eat into profits when accelerated depreciation is used.

Now, suppose that the office building you've invested in was put into service prior to 1981; you'd have a major plus. The old accelerated-depreciation rules would govern, and your gain from a sale would be taxed only to the extent that it exceeded straight-line depreciation.

Or suppose that the building houses rental apartments rather than offices. Because it's a residential property, only the difference between accelerated and straight-line depreciation would be recaptured.

There are dozens of other rules, most of them designed for tax specialists to decipher. But, clearly, Congress intended to steer investment dollars into residential real estate, as opposed to commercial and industrial properties, when it adopted the real-estate revisions included in the Economic Recovery Tax Act of 1981. Equally clear is the government's objective to discourage accelerated depreciation.

7

Some offers you can refuse

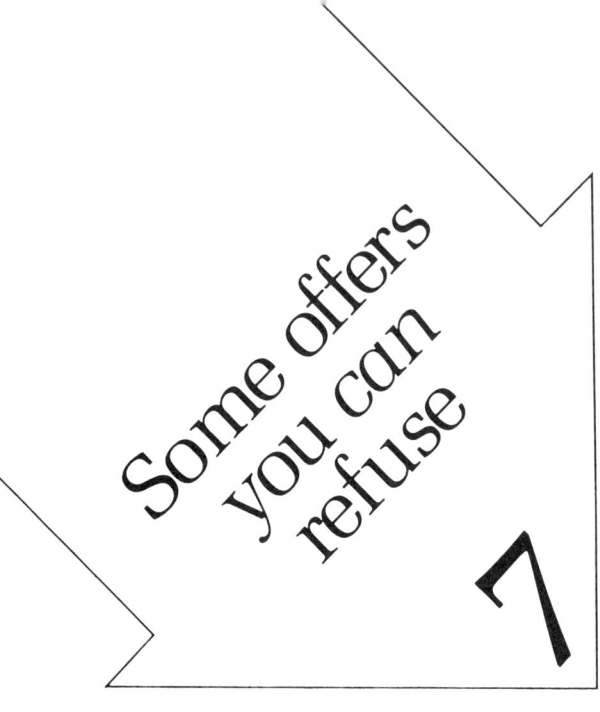

7 Some offers you can refuse

Be warned, especially if you're new to practice: Your profession conjures up a distinct image of a person with great money-making ability and very little time to think of anything other than work. To some, that's the image of an easy mark.

Undoubtedly, you'll be offered more than one deal "you can't afford to refuse." Some will be enticing indeed. Many will even be legitimate. But unless you've built up a thorough knowledge of investments or know where to go for advice, refuse. You can't afford not to.

Let's consider some examples—simplified by ignoring brokerage fees and tax consequences.

MARGIN ACCOUNTS

Let's say you've bought a few stocks and an eager broker sizes you up as ready for bigger things. He tells you that the stock of a maker of military electronic devices is down to an excellent buying range and the manufacturer has just been awarded a contract that will swell its earnings. The stock's now selling for 35, he says, giving you a chance to pick up 200 shares for $7,000 or so.

You like the idea and have confidence in the broker, but you protest that you can't come up with $7,000. "I'll gladly open a margin account for you," he answers. "Then for the 200 shares you'll put up only $3,500; we'll lend you the rest of the money."

You assume, of course, that the stock's price will climb several points, whereupon you'll sell and pay off your margin debt with profits fattened by leverage. Say the stock does rise to 45 from your price of 35. On 200 shares, that would represent a gain of $2,000, or 28.5 percent. But since you bought on margin, investing only half of the purchase price, your gain actually would be 57 percent.

Sounds great, doesn't it? And it is—except for one little detail: The stock has to rise in price. If instead it loses 10 points, dropping to 25, you're likely to receive a margin, or "maintenance," call. The broker will want more cash because the 100 shares that are, in effect, collateral for his $3,500 loan to you are now worth only $2,500, or 71 percent of the amount owed him. Regardless of changes in the stock's price, your margin debt to the broker remains $3,500, plus interest at the prevailing rate. So if you decided to sell when the stock was down 10 points, you'd be out $2,000 of your $3,500 investment—a 57 percent loss. Leverage, you see, magnifies losses just as effectively as it does gains.

That example deals with a 50 percent margin loan, a loan amounting to half the current market value of the stock being bought. The smaller the loan percentage, the greater the decline needed to trigger a margin call. Stock bought with only a 10 percent margin loan, for example, might decline to 15 percent or so of its purchase price before prompting a call for more money.

Some offers you can refuse

Margin requirements are closely supervised by the Federal Reserve Board, as well as by the exchanges, however, and—like the interest rates charged—fluctuate to reflect the prevailing economic conditions. A wildly churning bull market typically calls for the imposition of margin restraints: Investors might be required to put up 75 percent or more of the purchase price, for instance. Such restraints reduce trading activity and are viewed as safeguards for investors who tend to overreach when infected by bull-market exuberance.

SELLING SHORT

"He who sells what isn't his'n must pay it back or go to prison." That old stock market adage aptly describes the principal danger of selling short.

An investor sells a stock short because he expects its price to drop. Let's say you've been following a stock that's popular for shorting because its price typically swings rather widely in an active market. It's at 63, and you feel it's due for a fall. You don't own any of the stock, but you see a chance for profit in the downward price movement you expect. You place a short-sale order for, say, 200 shares—in effect borrowing from the broker the shares you're asking him to sell at 63.

If you've sized up the stock correctly and the price falls, say, to 53, you plan to buy 200 shares at that lower price. You'd use the cheaper shares to replace the shares you borrowed from your broker, "covering" your short position and walking away with a neat $10-per-share gain of $2,000.

The trouble is, it's no easier to be sure that a stock will fall than it is to accurately predict a rise. If, in our example, your stock's price should rise, you'd still owe your broker 200 shares. Having become one who'd sold "what isn't his'n," you'd have to buy those shares at the higher market price to repay him—and make up the loss out of your own pocket.

Obviously, shorting is a game for full-time tape watchers—the pros.

LETTER STOCK

Corporations issue stock, of course, to raise capital. Ordinarily an issue is underwritten by one or more investment bankers. They assure the corporation the cash it needs and hope to profit by marking up the price of the shares for resale.

Smaller corporations sometimes avoid that expensive procedure by issuing investment-letter stock—known simply as "letter" stock—that can't be readily resold. If the company is sound, with a promising product line, an offer of letter stock can fulfill every investor's dream: getting in on the ground floor of a hot new company. In addition, the stock—which has bypassed the underwriting process—can be bought at a fraction of the price it might ordinarily command.

There's nothing wrong with that—if everything works out. But consider: Letter stock represents mostly hope for an untried company. The stock has not been registered with the Securities and Exchange Commission and therefore cannot be sold on a public market. In fact, the "letter" you'd sign in buying it states that it is for "investment purposes only" and not for public resale. Such stock has no public market and little liquidity. If you want to sell, you must find a buyer privately or wait until the corporation registers the stock with the SEC for sale to the public.

Registration is what you're hoping for, of course. Then the shares you might have bought for pennies could very well be bid up to many times your purchase price. That could take years, though, even if all the hoped-for pluses fell into line. The risk that they won't fall into line, however, is substantial—too great for the inexperienced.

PUT AND CALL OPTIONS

An option is a contract that lets you sell (put) or buy (call) a stock at a certain price within a specified period of time. Some brokers insist that put and call options are conservative money-making devices that have been made safer than ever by the listing and public scrutiny provided by the Chicago Board Options Exchange and other exchanges. There's some merit to such thinking—if one assumes the investor fully understands options' uses. This very basic example shows that's not a logical assumption when it is applied to the typical beginning investor.

Let's say you like the stock of a supplier of oil-field needs and think its price will rise from 80 to perhaps 100 within six months. You could plunk down $8,000 and buy 100 shares now, but why tie up that money? Instead, a call option would let you buy the stock at 80 six months from now—even if the price has indeed risen to 100. You'd pay about $700 for that chance to profit later.

Six months later, let's say, the stock has hit your target of 100 and you exercise the call. You pay $8,000 for the 100 shares, making your total expenditure $8,700, and immediately sell them for $10,000. You've turned a profit of $1,300, and all you've invested is your option premium of $700. So your true gain would be a whopping 186 percent.

Suppose, however, that the stock's price does nothing, or even loses ground, during those six months. Obviously, you'd see no reason to exercise your call option. By not exercising it, you'd forfeit not only the $700 you paid for your option but also whatever amount the $700 might have earned had it been more gainfully employed.

Now let's put you on the other side of a call transaction. You're holding a block of that same stock for long-term appreciation. You sense a temporary weakness in it, though, and would like a hedge against a price drop. You decide to offer a put option for 100 shares at 80. A buyer picks up the six-month option for $7 a share. This gives you an immediate $700 gain to counter the price drop you fear.

But let's say your fears are groundless, and the stock rises. If it goes to 87, it will equal the buyer's $80 option purchase price plus the $7-per-share premium he paid for the call. That puts him on a clear track for profit, and he surely will exercise his option to buy your 100 shares. You'll still have your $700 gain, but you can't share in any further increase in the stock's price beyond 87.

Suppose you guessed correctly: The stock goes from 80 to 73. Your 100 shares show a paper loss of $700, but it's offset by the $700 option premium you received.

That's option trading at its most simplistic. We've spared you the complexities of option resales, buybacks, spreads, straddles, offsetting dividends, and similar recondite matters, knowledge of which can make put and call options lucrative—for the pros. Options are not for the beginning investor, but if they sound like something you'd like to grow into, ask your broker for booklets giving the more advanced course. If he can't oblige you, write to Public Investor Affairs, Chicago Board Options Exchange, Suite 2200, 141 W. Jackson Blvd., Chicago, Ill. 60604, requesting a copy of "Understanding Options." It's free. Or, if you'd like to explore options more fully, consult Chapter 10 for books you can purchase.

COMMODITY FUTURES

Those who put money into commodities—soybeans, pork bellies, sugar, that sort of thing—are called specula-

Some offers you can refuse

tors, not investors. That should tell you something. "Of all the ways of speculating," states a commodities handbook published by Merrill Lynch, Pierce, Fenner & Smith, "probably one of the most risky is speculating in commodity futures." Not only do futures prices move up and down rapidly, they are extremely sensitive to events that happen in every corner of the globe and at every hour of the day and night. Profits and losses resulting from these price gyrations are exaggerated by the especially high leverage of futures trading.

Volatile as it is, futures trading is vital to the economy. It provides a way for those who grow, process, or market farm products to lock in the price they need to turn a profit, even before the growing seasons begin. Speculators provide the risk capital required in return for a chance at big profits.

Futures are contracts for delivery of specified commodities at a later date. You might, for example, consider yourself an astute judge of coffee prices and, therefore, decide to investigate the potential for speculating. Let's say that coffee now sells for $2.03 a pound, but coffee futures for delivery in July are listed in your newspaper at 1.89^1/_2$. You believe the market has underestimated the expectation of increased production; the price, you think, more likely will be 1.84^1/_2$. So you put up $7,500 in margin money and sell a July contract at 1.89^1/_2$. That represents 37,500 pounds of coffee worth just over $71,000. Theoretically, if your estimate of 1.84^1/_2$ in July holds up, you'll gain 5 cents on each pound of coffee—a total of $1,875. Actually, you'll probably have settled for a fraction of that 25 percent gain on your margin investment and gone on to other trades long before July arrives. You certainly don't want to be holding that contract when the time comes for delivery.

It is the contracts that are traded, remember, not the actual coffee, cattle, wheat, or whatever. It is commonly estimated, in fact, that less than 3 percent of the commodities represented by traded contracts are ever actually delivered.

THOSE EXOTIC TAX SHELTERS

About the last offer you should accept as a beginning investor will probably be among the first made to you just because you're a doctor. It will be billed as a tax shelter, designed to appeal to that characteristic resident in every red-blooded American—the desire to decrease the amount of taxes owed.

But be wary. While properly designed tax shelters are legitimate and may serve you well, too many are designed to benefit only the plan's salesman and sponsor. All such plans, and especially the more exotic ones, demand the scrutiny of tax specialists.

Enough of that here; the mystique surrounding tax shelters is so powerful that the plans deserve chapters of their own.

Tax shelters: Looking before you leap 8

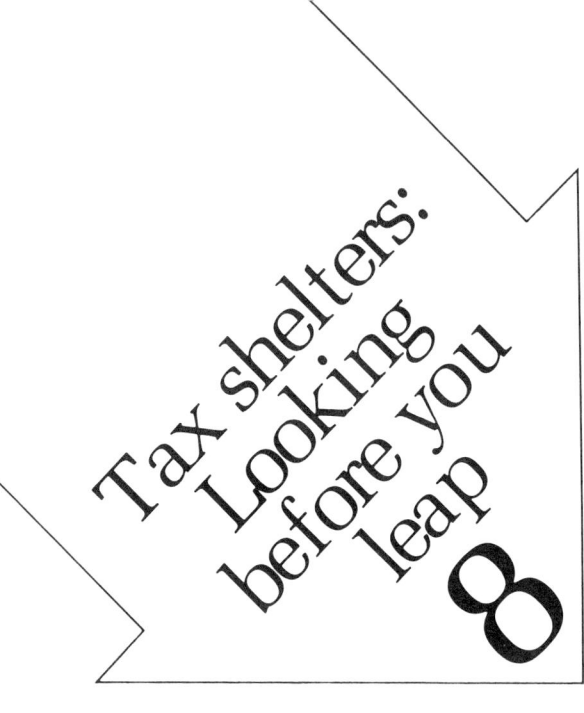

Tax shelters: Looking before you leap 8

"Sexy," in the jargon of the money world, means any action that generates excitement, activity, and high profits. The sexiest number to sashay down Wall Street in many a year is the tax shelter. How sexy is the tax shelter? In 1977, Merrill Lynch sold about $90 million worth, earning commissions of around $7 million. In 1980, the firm went over the half-billion dollar mark with commissions about six times greater than earlier. And that's just one company.

In 1981, however, Congress passed a sweeping tax-reduction package that stripped tax shelters of some of their allure. By repealing the extra tax on unearned income, Congress brightened the investment climate and removed a big incentive to seek shelter. Still, despite reform, tax shelters—while rarely well understood—continue to attract high-level earners. Wall Street and independent promoters are searching high and low for everything they can possibly represent as a tax-shelter deal. The deal that would languish if called venture capital has a powerful allure for investors when called a tax shelter. Unfortunately, however, there are many more salesmen out there than there are solid deals worth your money and effort.

WHAT ACTUALLY IS A TAX SHELTER?

A tax-exempt municipal bond is a tax shelter, although almost never called by that name. So are the Individual Retirement Accounts (IRAs), which since 1982 have allowed any wage earner to sock away as much as $2,000 a year on a tax-deferred basis.

In common usage, however, most tax shelters are limited partnerships. Those designing the deal and proposing to oversee it usually become the general partners. Investors recruited to buy into it become limited partners. For you as an investor, this means just what it says: Your responsibility for losses and liabilities is limited to the extent of your investment. Similarly, you share proportionately in any profits and tax credits.

Even before Congress repealed the tax on unearned income, some sophisticated financial writers were claiming there's actually no such thing as a tax shelter, merely good and bad investments. If you are able to accept that simple statement, you may save yourself a lot of money and grief.

In creating so-called tax shelters, Congress's intent was, in the words of Marvin Kamensky, a Chicago attorney specializing in taxes, "to push money into areas where the infusion of capital benefits the economy or serves a socially useful purpose." The intent was not to help rich people avoid taxes, but to provide incentives to put money into risky but necessary undertakings that would not be acceptable in a conservative investment program. In fact, "You enter into the tax shelter knowing that you're doing something common business sense would tell you not to do," says Peter Deiro, senior trust officer of Chemical Bank in New York City.

The IRS says you must go into a shelter seeking a profit, but common sense says you have to be able to absorb the loss. Don't waste your time with anyone who tries to sell you tax benefits instead of a program with a reasonable chance of showing an eventual decent profit. *Always determine the economic upside*, advises Jerome R. Rosenberg, Manhattan tax attorney and financial writer. You just can't get rich losing money. If there is no likelihood of any profit other than a tax break, he says, you can bet the IRS will disallow your shelter. The deal may have been put together by perfectly reputable professionals, but read all their literature with a jaundiced eye. If their prospectus says, "The IRS might hold ...," it's just as likely that the IRS will not hold—and you'll be left holding the bag.

In shelters other than purely tax-exempt investments, such as municipal bonds, you do not avoid income tax; you simply defer paying it. Or, in the very best tax shelters, you convert high-bracket income into lower-bracket income.

Deferring taxes is, in effect, borrowing money from Uncle Sam—and that's not bad. If that borrowed money is left to work for you on a tax-deferred basis—as in an IRA—the interest and dividends it generates compound to the fullest. Money that ordinarily would have gone for taxes is left working for you.

A day of reckoning does come, of course. Typically, any shelter based on tax deferment can be liquidated when you reach age $59^1/_2$. You *must* start drawing from it—and paying taxes on those withdrawals—at age $70^1/_2$. Still, you will have had the benefit of tax-free compounding. And, presumably, your takedown of funds will not begin until you've retired and entered a reduced tax bracket.

WHO SHOULD—AND SHOULD NOT—GET INTO TAX SHELTERS?

There's an acid test to decide the point at which you might reasonably consider exploring tax shelters. It suggests that any beginning investor whose income is not taxed at the highest marginal rate should avoid the shelter game. Furthermore, like many other experienced tax practitioners and reputable broker-dealers, Jerome Rosenberg recommends sheltering only that portion of income that's subject to the highest tax rate—i.e., only income above $85,600 for those filing joint returns.

"In an equity-oriented deal such as oil and gas or real estate," says Lawrence J. Winston, senior vice president of E.F. Hutton & Co., "most brokerage houses will insist that an investor be paying tax at the 40 to 50 percent marginal rate and have liquid assets of at least $100,000, not counting his home and cars. In an equipment-leasing program, which has the highest requirements, he has to . . . have assets of $150,000 to $200,000." And if you're worried about meeting college expenses for your kids, a responsible broker will tell you to try something else.

Liquidity is a major concern, which is why good brokers want you to have substantial assets to fall back on if need be. Shelters are notoriously illiquid, especially real estate and other forms that have hefty up-front deductions. Liquidity can also be a problem when you hold an interest in a limited partnership, since the general partner's approval is usually required before you can transfer your share of the shelter.

You may also need backup funds; it's not unusual for partners to be asked for extra payments to keep a program going during a dry spell or recession. Here lies the danger of throwing good money after bad—pumping more and more dollars into a losing business, thereby increasing your potential (or actual) losses.

It should always be *your* individual situation that finally determines what you should do. Most people who have just begun to hit the big-time bracket shouldn't jump the gun on shelters. But if you're single—or married with a high dual income and intend not to have children—and you can foresee no great capital needs within the next five or 10 years, you might risk a tax shelter. Or if you know that for one year only, for whatever reason, you'll have a huge jump in income that won't continue, you might consider a shelter, but you really owe it to yourself to exhaust other avenues first.

In other words, it's the rare beginning investor who should be spending time and money on shelters. Unfortunately, shelter fever is epidemic in the medical community. It could even be called iatrogenic, since doctors are doing a great job of infecting themselves and each other. And if the most discouraging words don't inoculate you, you'll probably have to develop immunity through painful contact.

That happened to Vernon A. Ingle, a general practitioner in Montebello, Calif. "I'm lucky to have lost only about $15,000," he says. "Tax shelters are a joke, and I mean a sick joke." He got into three ventures, including one that just couldn't lose: owning U.S. post office buildings and leasing them to the government. But it did lose, thanks to misfortune and poor planning. "I was a dummy," Ingle says. "I've learned, I hope. I consider the $15,000 I lost to be my tuition."

RESISTING THOSE SALES PITCHES

It's difficult for doctors to avoid tax-shelter propositions. You're simply in a high-risk category. You're likely to hear about deals in three ways: solicitation, professional advice, and homework. Only the advice of professionals you trust and your own painstaking study are relatively safe. Management consultant Nelson Young of Fort Lauderdale observes: "It's understandably hard even for the cautious doctor not to be impressed when he hears colleagues in the hospital cafeteria—who rarely air their investment disasters—bragging about those good deals they're into. But the fact that a lot of people are going into a deal doesn't mean it's a good one. It does usually mean that there's a tremendous sales effort under way."

Make no mistake: The competition for doctors' investment dollars is fierce. Promoters hire bright, articulate salespeople—women as well as men—who are trained in subtle and not-so-subtle methods of overcoming every form of sales resistance but a flat "no." These people operate on two basic principles: (1) Every doctor wants into a tax shelter and (2) all's fair provided it doesn't violate the letter of the law. However, as you know, not every doctor should have a tax shelter and, when it comes to the law, the IRS is just as concerned with the spirit as with the letter.

When you're approached, always ask yourself, "Why me?" Let's say you're an internist in Ohio and you get a breathless call or an ardent, unsolicited letter inviting you to join an orange-growing shelter in California. Are you going to ask yourself if all the internists in California have just experienced a sudden serious drop in income? Otherwise, why would the promoter go so far afield to find you and other takers?

Turn a deaf ear to anyone saying that your name came from an exclusive list of sophisticated investors (it very likely came from an AMA directory). Show your sophistication by dismissing that spiel. The farther the shelter from your area and expertise, the more likely that the promoter will take the money and run.

There's often a near deadline for these offerings. The "last day" to get in on the deal is Tuesday morning, when this is already Friday afternoon. If you don't have the time to investigate the deal thoroughly, let it pass. There'll be another offer tomorrow. Count on it.

Christmas, by the way, is usually quite wonderful for promoters because so many people decide in December that they needed a shelter yesterday. The seriously rich who work at maintaining and increasing their money hate surprises. Unless an obscure uncle—perhaps a tea planter in up-country Sri Lanka—dies and leaves an unexpected bequest, they want to know exactly how much they are going to make, spend, pay in taxes, and invest. They don't make their decisions in December, nor should you.

Remember also that the money that supports this scatter-gun approach comes out of funds that could have gone into the project itself. If you get involved, a good part of your investment could go to pay the costs of soliciting hundreds of other doctors who did not. So be suspicious of slick, color brochures, lavish hospitality suites, and WATS-line phone calls.

WHOSE ADVICE CAN YOU TRUST?

Doctors are as prone as anyone else to the mystique of "professionalism." Be wary of a promoter who says he'd prefer to discuss the technical details with your lawyer or accountant because it's easier for one financial professional to talk to another. That probably means that a nice little piece of the action is about to be shared with the very person most likely to know your weak spot. If you are sophisticated enough to get involved in tax shelters, you are sophisticated enough to be dealt with as an investor whose intelligence—by the mere fact of your having been certified in medicine—is at least a considerable notch or two above average.

If you have found a trustworthy adviser, *trust* him or her, especially when you're told that the deal is *not* for you. Nelson Young tells of a client, a young doctor who was short of money, who was approached to sink cash into a cattle deal that would save him $15,000 in taxes that very year.

"Well," said Young, "I pointed out to the doctor that his financial picture didn't justify a $60,000 obligation. He still wanted to do it, so I brought in his attorney for a meeting with the salesman. The salesman was too savvy to argue when I explained why this was premature for our client. He said, 'That's an ultraconservative position, but I understand your point of view.'

"We left thinking our doctor would drop out of the deal. But when I checked in at his office several months later, I learned he was in up to his stethoscope. The salesman, who had helped the doctor concoct a fictitious net-worth statement, cheerfully justified his activities to me with this candid admission: 'You'd look at the whole deal differently if you'd earned $9,000 for six hours of conversation the way I did.'"

Be inclined to distrust any adviser who gets a commission or bonus if you invest. That person will not be disinterested. Unfortunately, there's nothing unusual about a promoter's paying a lawyer or accountant 10 to 15 percent of whatever amount you are persuaded to put up—even though that, in the view of Stephen L. Hammerman, New York Regional Administrator for the SEC, constitutes fraud on the investor. If your adviser does take a commission, this should be disclosed to you. Every commission paid means that much less money actually invested. You pay for the advice twice over, first as your fee to your lawyer or accountant, and a second time as the commission he pockets for parting you from your money.

A 10 or 15 percent commission may not seem a terribly serious matter, just the cost of doing business. But let's look at a real case—one where there's no evidence that the company and the people involved were anything less than reputable. A drilling fund set forth its prospectus in 100 pages densely packed with arcane information. The deal solicited $40 million, of which $5 million went immediately into commissions and management fees, and $200,000 into organizing fees. That left $34.8 million for actual drilling, still quite a tidy sum. But translated into financial realities, that means a front load of 13 percent.

In the five years before the deal, that same company had found $350 million in investments. How much cash was actually distributed to the limited partners? $7.4 million. But the general partner (a company) got $17 million in management fees over that same time span! Such revenues boosted their stock by 15 percent in the last three years of that same period.

That company looks philanthropic when compared with another high-figure deal. The general partner put up 1 percent of the many millions required, while the limited partners put up 99 percent. (Remember that stockholders have some say in management and policy, but limited partners have none.) *If* there are any earnings, they will be split 90-10 until the limited partners just make back their investments in cash and tax write-offs. Then the limited partners' share will fall to 60 percent of profits, while the general partner, with his 1 percent no longer at risk, will reap 40 percent. And the inequity doesn't stop there. Only 90 percent of the money from the limited partners went into the business itself, while the audacious general partner received 10 percent to cover "various expenses."

Shares in a limited partnership constitute securities and, as such, must be either exempt or registered with the SEC. Unless you're well versed in this complex field, regard any obscurity about registration as a tipoff to fraud of some kind. If the shares are registered, there must be a prospectus. Read it—and don't hesitate to keep asking questions until you get satisfactory answers. If there are commissions or hefty "management fees" or "organizing expenses" involved, the prospectus should disclose them.

THE LURE OF THE EXOTICS

Tax shelters are divided into two groups: the exotics and the decent shots. There are two kinds of exotics: the obviously far-out and the outwardly ordinary. Some exotic tax shelters follow the letter of the law but don't stand up in court, while others fit the law like a glove but are dubious investments nevertheless. Shelters have recently been offered in manuscripts, lithographic plates, and master recordings. An advertisement in *The Wall Street Journal* even offered a 3:1 write-off featuring Bibles for missionaries.

The incentive most of these exotic deals offer is an investment tax credit. To spur investment in business assets (not real estate, however), the IRS may allow you to deduct as much as 10 percent of your investment from your income tax—*not* your taxable income—during the first year. This tax credit is a bonus to you, pure and simple, from Uncle Sam. In the case of a 3:1 write-off, the promoter promises you leverage so that you are able to deduct $3 from your income tax for every $1 of your own money you ante up. However, the IRS has a distinct tendency to look askance at offbeat deals involving high credits on small investments. When your investment tax credit is disallowed, you get to pay the IRS back, dollar for dollar.

Here's an illustration of another exotic tax shelter—one that's legal but a dubious investment. A promoter offered a new process for the manufacture of bleach through alternative energy sources, which meant an alternative-energy tax credit of $6,000. The deal required a minimum investment of $10,000 cash with a $20,000 note with recourse (you would be personally responsible for the amount of the note even if the project failed). Bleach hardly seems exotic. But what do you know about its manufacture? Or about alternative sources of energy? Would you risk a hefty $30,000 investment to buy stock in such an enterprise? Not likely, unless you have specialized knowledge that makes this bet a relatively sure thing. Just because it's called a tax shelter is no reason to suspend the rules of sound investment. In fact, this offer is a very risky investment with a tax credit as the rather small cherry on top.

Chapter 9 explores some legitimate tax shelters. But as you read about the money it's possible to make (and save), please don't forget all the warning signs posted in the chapter you've just read.

They boil down to a sound maxim reputable financial advisers swear by: No tax shelter is worth its salt unless it is first of all a good investment.

Tax shelters: Playing to win in a risky game

9

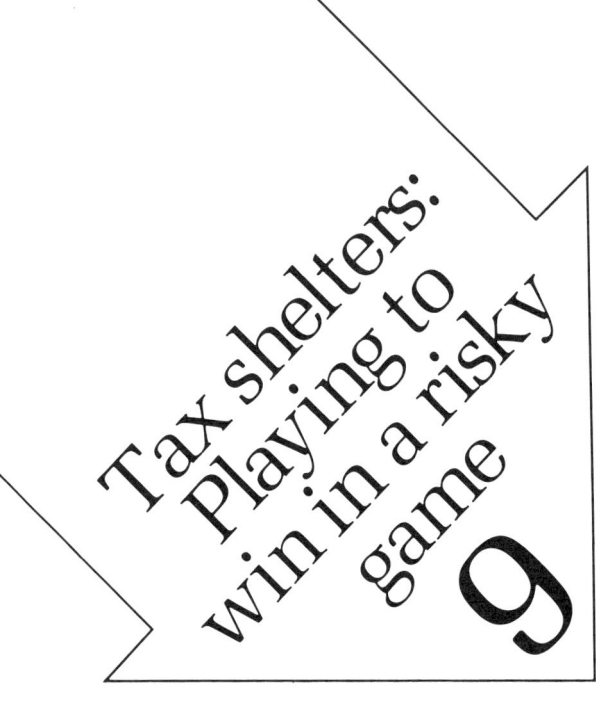

9. Tax shelters: Playing to win in a risky game

Just about everybody concedes that taxes are necessary in a civilized society. Just about everybody, too, resents having to pay them—especially those taxes on income, which seem to penalize us for being productive members of society.

It's only human nature, then, that we seek ways to minimize the taxes we pay. And it's only natural that the Internal Revenue Service, charged with collecting our taxes, seeks ways to maximize them.

That dichotomy has led over the years to a Tom-and-Jerry routine so stylized that it might well have been choreographed: The Treasury (with Congressional help) imposes tax laws; we taxpayers (with tax-attorney help) find loopholes in them; the IRS closes those loopholes; we find more; it closes them; we find more, etc.

It's all legitimate; the IRS insists it doesn't want us paying more in taxes than the laws say we should. It expects us to use all possible legal channels to reduce them. And we, in return, expect to pay heavy penalties if the IRS or the U.S. Tax Court can prove that we've stepped outside legal bounds.

It isn't surprising that within recent history Congress has enacted the Tax Reform Act of 1969, the Tax Reduction Act of 1975, the Revenue Act of 1978, the Windfall Profit Tax Act of 1980, the Economic Recovery Tax Act of 1981, and the Tax Equity and Fiscal Responsibility Act of 1982—all of which were designed, in part, to make tax shelters less attractive.

Nor is it surprising that the Supreme Court sided with the IRS and Director Philip E. Coates in mid-1983 in their battle to eliminate tax shelters that they consider "abusive."

What's abusive? When a shelter involves transactions with little or no economic substance, when its claimed tax benefits are disproportionate to its economic benefits, Coates says, that's abusive. Abuses might range from a rather common one (and therefore one you should guard against) of overvaluation—in which promoters pump up a shelter's stated values in order to provide inflated write-offs—to fictitious transactions, backdated documents, and reporting of nonexistent assets.

Citing the growth in tax shelters, as well as the rise in shelter "abuses," the director said that in 1973, when the IRS first began to probe shelters seriously, auditors examined only about 400 tax returns involving them. Just 10 years later, he said, almost 325,000 shelter returns were being examined. Worse, some 16,300 cases, involving more than $1 billion in tax deficiencies, were pending before the Tax Court.

Penalties, too, have been stepped up. Consider, for example, those for overvaluation of the property being invested in: A 1981 ruling set penalties of 10 percent, added to the tax underpayment, if the property was overvalued by 150 to 200 percent; 20 percent, plus the underpayment, if overvaluation runs to 200 to 250 percent, and 30 percent, added to the underpaid amount, for overvaluations above 250 percent.

For abuses other than overvaluation, a 1982 tax law imposes an alternative penalty: If you understate your tax by 10 percent or $5,000, whichever is greater, you'll pay an additional tax of 10 percent of the understatement. Of course, you'll be charged interest at going rates on the amount underpaid.

The new rules can trip you up without your even being aware of violations. That's because the IRS now may audit tax-shelter partnerships before approaching the individual partners. If the partnership is found at fault, you as an individual partner have virtually no defense.

But, given the persistence and ingenuity of tax attorneys, and despite the whittling away of their advantages, tax shelters still live.

There are tax-shelter investments to be had in such diverse areas as cattle feeding and Broadway plays, tree farming and Thoroughbred racehorses. Many of them are relatively risky, however, and too demanding of time and money to be of interest to beginning investors. So we'll stick here to the three types of shelters that seem to be most favored by doctors: real estate, energy exploration, and equipment leasing.

As with most other types of shelters, you probably shouldn't consider these unless you're solidly in the top marginal tax bracket. And remember this baleful advice from Leonard Bailin, a New York City-based attorney and tax-shelter specialist: "The time to decide how to get out of a shelter is when you buy in."

REAL ESTATE

You can use almost any form of real-estate investment to achieve tax savings; but chances are that the type of shelter you'll encounter most often will be a limited-partnership syndication, as described in the previous chapter.

Just bear in mind that real estate—like all other investments with tax-shelter propensities—is constantly being scrutinized by the IRS for possible abuses.

Just a few years ago, limited-partnership participations were sold only by salesmen who handled nothing else, or by a few enterprising real-estate dealers. Some still are. But now, the same brokerage firm that might sell you stocks and bonds will be happy to sell you a limited-partnership participation; and it'll be one the firm's own real-estate specialists have checked out and found to pass muster.

Such sales are known as public offerings. They probably will be made nationwide, and the properties in which they invest partners' funds may be scattered over several states. The cost of a participation may be as low as $5,000 or $10,000.

As a high-profile professional, however, you're just as likely to be offered an opportunity to invest as a limited partner in an office building that's to be constructed just down the street, or in a shopping center on your town's outskirts. That would be a private offering, one likely to be made only to local investors. The cost of a limited partnership in such a real-estate package typically would be much higher, perhaps in the $50,000 to $100,000 range.

There are countless other ways to invest in real estate, not the least of which is simply to buy an income-producing property and look after it yourself. The limited partnerships provide the cleanest investment route, however, for the busy investor who prefers to let his money work while he pursues his career.

Taxes—which both giveth and taketh away—are a primary ingredient in all real-estate investments, whatever their form. Even if you're investing with a general partner you know you can trust, you'd be wise to seek the counsel of a good accountant and a tax-savvy attorney.

Real-estate investments can get into big money. And tax laws can be very complex, not to mention fast-changing.

Let's say, for example, that in January 1982 you paid $50,000 for a 1/24 share of a privately offered $6 million shopping-center deal. Of the $6 million, $1.2 million came from investors' cash and $4.8 million was provided as a mortgage loan from a bank. Your share of the $4.8 million debt, $200,000, is on a nonrecourse basis—meaning that you don't have to repay it if the venture fails. Tax laws now let you capitalize that $200,000 along with your $50,000 cash outlay, which means you can depreciate $250,000 while laying out only $50,000—a 4-to-1 write-off, in other words.

If that sounds like too good a deal, take note that the IRS agrees with you—and if it gets the backing it seeks from the Supreme Court, recapture rules undoubtedly will be imposed to water down still another tax shelter's attributes. Note, too, that for purposes of simplification, examples used here will ignore the portion of an investment that goes toward buying land, since—as we've pointed out—land cannot be depreciated.

Real property not for residential use is to be depreciated over 15 years, says the Tax Act of 1981. That same act provides that all accelerated depreciation—now called ACRS (for accelerated cost recovery system) depreciation—on nonresidential properties will be subject to recapture when you sell your share of the venture.

A shopping center is nonresidential, of course, so your partnership very likely will choose to depreciate the property using a straight-line write-off—$1/_{15}$ of the total each year. Your $250,000 investment then yields an annual deduction of $16,667 from your taxable income. In the highest marginal tax bracket, you'd save a total of $25,000 in federal income tax through 1984.

Now let's say you want to sell your share of the shopping-center project at the end of 1984, even though you could have continued to shelter your income for another 12 years. Since straight-line depreciation isn't subject to recapture, you'd get to keep the entire $25,000 (under present tax rules). And any profit you'd make on the sale of your investment would be taxed at the 20 percent capital-gains rate.

What if you'd bought into a residential property instead of a commercial one? Because the Government wants to encourage growth in housing, you'd find recapture rules more lenient. Using the same example, let's assume that your partnership takes advantage of those rules and applies ACRS depreciation, writing off 175 percent of the declining balance (that means reducing each year's undepreciated balance by 175 percent of the amount straight-line depreciation would have permitted). Your tax saving in this case would total $43,750 for the three years, a hefty increase over the $25,000 that straight-line depreciation would have permitted.

Now suppose that property is low-income subsidized housing under construction. A whole new set of tax rules would apply. The investment property might qualify for 200 percent declining-balance depreciation. You might also be able to deduct the full amount of mortgage interest and taxes—all taxes—incurred during the first year, or "construction period," instead of spreading them over the 15-year life of the investment. Those features combine to make low-income subsidized housing an excellent shelter.

But let's be realistic: The search-and-destroy mission launched against tax shelters by the IRS places all tax-saving measures in jeopardy. We know that starting in 1985—unless tax-attorney diligence comes through again—all accelerated depreciation of real estate will be ended; all depreciation reverts to the straight-line basis. It's practically a certainty, too, that the balance of a nonrecourse loan will be taxed when the property to which it was applied is sold. In the case of the foregoing examples, that would mean your $200,000 share of the loan would be taxed as a gain. It becomes imperative, in other words, that you go over any proposed real-estate investment with your accountant and attorney, as well as with any real-estate specialist whose opinions you value; rules of the game are changing constantly.

There are other risks to be considered when dealing in real properties. A commercial tenant could suffer business reverses, leaving your partnership with a lease that's either in default or litigation. Property taxes might be raised unexpectedly. Misforecast traffic patterns could leave your property sitting outside the mainstream. If the shelter's property is foreclosed, you're liable for the recapture of depreciation you've taken on it. You might even find yourself paying tax on a paper profit, which is what happens when a promoter overstates a property's value.

As an example, let's say a promoter buys an apartment house for $5 million and unloads it on the tax-shelter partnership for $6 million. Along with 19 other investors, you buy 1/20 of the shares at a cost of $50,000. That $1 million in cash goes into the promoter's pocket, and the shelter undertakes a $5 million mortgage for the rest.

The IRS, however, can figure the property's true market value at $5 million and cut back all depreciation write-offs based on the bloated $6 million price. We'll say that the IRS accepts the $6 million figure, but the burden placed on the partnership by the inflated mortgage creates a cash shortage. The limited partners, protected by their nonrecourse agreement, refuse to put up the additional money needed to keep the venture afloat. The partnership defaults on the mortgage, and the building is foreclosed.

The IRS treats the foreclosure exactly as if the shelter had sold the building to the lender for the outstanding balance of the mortgage. Let's assume that the balance is $4.5 million at the time of foreclosure, and that your group by then has written off $2 million on the deal. The IRS adds that $2 million to the $4.5 million "selling price," subtracts the original $6 million cost, and finds that the shelter "gained" $500,000. That, of course, is money you never saw—and money that never existed, except on paper. Yet, you must pay tax on your share of that mythical profit, at unearned-income rates.

You can avoid such inflated deals. "Ask to see the real-estate contracts and other actual documents that were the basis of the promises made in the offering circular," advises Chicago attorney Marvin Kamensky. "Then you can tell how much the price of the building was kited and how much equity went to the promoter. If the promoter refuses to show you the documents, forget the deal." If the venture involves construction of a single building, ask a local bank's construction-loan officer what typical costs per square foot have been for similar buildings. If the promoter's projected construction costs seem out of line, the deal might be too risky.

It's to your advantage that the promoter have a substantial, if not major, interest in the shelter. If he takes up-front money only, he isn't motivated to see the venture through a profitable lifetime. He's more likely to live up to his responsibilities as a general partner if he has a hefty portion of the deal. "Some investors think they've made a smart deal when they squeeze the promoter's share down, says attorney Leonard Bailin. "That's not smart. It just places the promoter in a position to take what he can and let the shelter slide."

Finally, any real-estate tax shelter must reckon with the vagaries of the real-estate market. Will there ever again be an era of rapid appreciation like that brought on by inflated building costs and high interest rates from, roughly, 1978 to 1982? For the good of the overall economy, we should hope not. "But," says Henry Von Kohorn, a Westport, Conn., consultant on real-estate financing, "quality income-producing properties will continue to go up in value. The investor must do the legwork to make sure, however, that he is getting quality."

EQUIPMENT LEASING

With the Economic Recovery Tax Act of 1981, Congress leaned over backward to make equipment leasing both safe and attractive. However, this type of shelter still typically requires a large cash outlay and is not for the small investor.

You can buy and lease out almost any expensive durable equipment. Your best bet is a durable asset that's likely to remain valuable when the lease period expires. (For lease period, in effect, read "write-off" or "recovery period"—the number of years over which the law allows you to depreciate your investment.) Airplanes, barges, freight cars, and computers are favorite shelters.

Three characteristics add to the attractiveness of equipment leasing:

▶ End-of-the-lease purchase agreement. Before signing the lease, you (the lessor) and the actual user of the equipment (the lessee) negotiate the price at which the lessee will buy the equipment from you when the lease expires. This means you won't have to worry about disposing of the airplane, computer, or whatever after several years of wear and tear. Make the lessee responsible for maintenance and repair, and insure the equipment against damage or destruction.

▶ Fast write-off. There are four "classes" of equipment, each of which may be depreciated over various periods of time. For present purposes, we're interested only in the three-, five-, and 10-year classes (see Box 9-1, pages 120-121). In addition, you may choose to use the straight-line method or the ACRS method; as with real estate, the ACRS method can be used only until 1985, and recapture applies if the lease is transferred before the recovery period expires (Box 9-1). If you elect ACRS, you'd use 150 percent of the declining balance and switch in 1985 to a method called sum-of-years-digits.

Notice the special three-year write-off advantage available to lessors of equipment used for research and development—an advantage partly offset, however, by a smaller investment tax credit.

▶ The investment tax credit. It's widely assumed that equipment leasing qualifies you for an investment tax credit. This is not necessarily true. A limited partnership or individual who does not satisfy certain IRS requirements cannot get the credit. For example, all three parties to a leasing venture—the lessor, the lessee, and the financing provider—must specify that the lease is a "safe harbor" lease. There are other legal niceties that can trip you up, so it's important to get expert advice before putting up a hefty cash investment in the expectation of a tax credit.

The investment tax credit is limited to a percentage of the amount you have "at risk": 6 percent for three-year property, 10 percent for all other classes. "At risk" applies to your actual cash outlay and to money you've borrowed for the venture. If the lender meets certain legal requirements, even a nonrecourse loan may be considered "at risk." To reap this bonanza, however, you must be *actually* at risk for at least 20 percent of the total cost of the property, or "basis."

Suppose, for example, you put $200,000 down on a $1 million fleet of tractor-trailers and sign an $800,000 nonrecourse note. Ordinarily, you'd receive a tax credit of 10 percent of the $200,000 for which you're actually at risk, or $20,000. But since you've put up at least 20 percent of the "basis" in cash, the tax credit is based on the entire

BOX 9-1

Tax treatment of classes of leased equipment

Class	Kinds of equipment	Straight-line recovery options	Tax credit
3-year property	Autos, light trucks, equipment used in research and development	3, 5, or 12 years	6%
5-year property	Most machinery and equipment, agricultural structures, petroleum-storage facilities	5, 12, or 25 years	10
10-year property	Certain public-utility equipment, theme and amusement park properties, railroad tank cars, mobile homes, coal-utilization property	10, 25, or 35 years	10
15-year property	Long-lived public-utility machinery and facilities	15, 35, or 45 years	10

$1 million. You receive $100,000—and if the venture fails, you're out only the $200,000 you anted up. Remember, though, that the IRS looks askance at nonrecourse loans; and if the courts uphold its view, your share of the loan would be taxed as a gain upon sale of the shelter property.

Here's a very simplified sketch of how an equipment-leasing shelter might work: We'll assume that in 1982 you and three other investors were brought together in a limited partnership structured to qualify for the investment tax credit. For $50,000 in cash and a 20 percent,

Recapture of ACRS in excess of straight-line recovery over	Recapture of tax credit if sold before				
	1 year	2 years	3 years	4 years	5 years
5 years	100%	66%	33%	—	—
8 years	100	80	60	40%	20%
15 years	100	80	60	40	20
22 years	100	80	60	40	20

$100,000 nonrecourse note each, you and your partners bought $600,000 worth of new machinery to be used in electronics research.

Since you're allowed to write off your investment in three years (in effect, it's four), you don't need to use ACRS depreciation; you use the straight-line method. That gives you a tax deduction of $25,000 in 1982; $50,000 in 1983; another $50,000 in 1984; and $25,000 again in 1985, according to the tax law passed in 1981. In the highest marginal tax bracket, you'd save roughly $75,000 in taxes. No one partner is actually at risk for as much as 20 percent of the entire cost of the machinery; so your investment tax credit is limited to 6 percent of your cash investment, or $3,000. Add that to your tax saving, and you reap a total of $78,000 on a $50,000 cash investment.

You and your partners sign a four-year lease at $90,000 a year with the company that will use the machinery. The user also agrees to pay the partnership $400,000 for the machinery at the end of the four-year lease. Split four ways, this gives you a cash income of $22,500 for the first four years and a $100,000 long-term capital gain in the fifth year.

Offsetting this income, the tax saving on depreciation, and the investment tax credit is a whopping $35,000 annual debt service. Retiring that $100,000 debt will be your biggest hurdle. During the first year, the investment tax credit will let you just about break even on a cash basis. The higher write-off allowed you during the next two years will enable you to look at some folding money: about $6,000 in 1983 and $5,000 in 1984. Keep some of it for 1985, though, when the reduced write-off—not offset by a tax credit this time—will take about $5,000 away from you.

It's the fifth year, with its guaranteed sale of the machinery, that will be golden. Your only deductible expense will be the interest portion of the $35,000 loan repayment. (To avoid recapture, you couldn't sell before fully depreciating the investment.) The net income—$85,000—is taxed at only the long-term capital-gains rate. You'll end up with a five-year after-tax profit of over 100 percent on your $50,000 investment, or 20 percent each year.

This very simplified example exposes some of the pitfalls of equipment leasing. First, the investment tax credit: It's not always what it's cracked up to be. Second, the loan: A short payback and high interest rate can virtually wipe out your cash profit. Third, the profit itself: Not terribly spectacular except in comparison with the two lean and two only-slightly-plump years preceding it. If we've painted a bleaker picture of equipment leasing than you've seen in promotional literature, it's because this kind of tax shelter can batter an investor who doesn't have a thick cushion of cash to fall back on.

ENERGY EXPLORATION

For our purposes, this means drilling for oil and gas. Nuclear fission and coal are controversial; anyhow, they don't provide the attractive tax benefits that drilling for oil and gas does. Geothermal energy, although it's been running Italy's railroads and heating much of Paris for many years, hasn't yet caught on in the U.S. It would still be classified as an exotic investment and, without clear tax breaks, would not be worth the risk unless you're eager to lose money.

Popular guides to investing in oil and gas abound. They tend to be full of terms like "mud," "footage," "turnkey," "casing point," and "thermal recovery." Read several pieces of literature to make sure of a consensus on what such terms mean—and quiz the promoter to make sure of mutual understanding. (If you're buying into a drilling program via a brokerage house, ask to speak with the petroleum analyst. It can be worth the long-distance call. Your local "customer's man" is unlikely to know much about this field unless you live in oil- and gas-producing territory.)

In passing the Economic Recovery Tax Act of 1981, Congress didn't slight investors in oil and gas exploration when it handed out the tax breaks. Royalty owners—as investors in drilling are called—received a $2,500 credit against windfall-profits tax in 1981. Instead of a flat tax credit, royalty owners can claim an exemption against the windfall-profits tax equal to the proceeds on two barrels a day for oil produced in 1982, 1983, and 1984, and three barrels a day from 1985 on. Barrels translate into dollars this way: At a conservative $30 per barrel before tax, 720 barrels per year are worth $21,600. At the 1982 windfall-profits tax rate of 27.5 percent, that's equivalent to a tax credit of $5,940.

As the exemption mounts, the windfall-profits tax declines: from 25 percent in 1983 to 22.5 percent in 1984, 20 percent in 1985, and 15 percent from 1986 on. This means an effective tax credit of 180 barrels per year in 1983, 162 in 1984, 216 in 1985, and 162 in 1986 and after. (The big jump in 1985 is due to the switch in exemption from two to three barrels—an attractive investment opportunity if you're willing to take the risk.)

The depletion allowance hasn't dried up, either, although it is being cut back—from 20 percent in 1981 to 15 percent beginning in 1984.

You can invest either in exploration—wildcatting in fresh territory to find new resources—or in development of known fields. Development, of course, is less risky than exploration, and the cost to investors is correspondingly greater and the potential return less—rarely more than 2:1. Either way, a private drilling program is likely to return more than a public one, and a limited partnership is preferable to a joint venture. In a joint venture, you may be held individually liable for the project's entire expenses—a disaster if there's an oil spill, for example. If you want to invest heavily in oil and gas—not ordinarily a wise move for a beginner—dilute your risk by spreading your money over several projects.

Between 65 and 90 percent of the cost of drilling and completing a well is "intangible"; it consists of labor and other elements that have no salvage value. These intangible costs can be written off in the year they're incurred—the first year of the program. You're then allowed an investment tax credit on the tangible costs. This means a big first-year deduction from your taxable income. If the well is productive, you can continue to write off the depletion allowance. "Lifting costs," or the expense of getting the oil from the ground to the refinery, further decrease your taxable income. But even with all these deductions from income, it's possible for a productive well to pay back your investment in as little as three years.

What if the well is dry? That's the risk you take. You can still write off those intangible drilling expenses, however. And the prospectus should stipulate that the general partner must return the money you put up for completing the well, drill a replacement well, or otherwise protect your investment in case the well is dry. However, the risk is significant—in fact, oil and gas exploration is considered the most speculative kind of legitimate investment.

You can minimize your risk by carefully checking the promoter's track record and by reading prospectuses. You should also pay attention to what happens if the drill strikes gas instead of oil: Does the prospectus promise a pipeline hookup? Finally, the time of year is important. If the first 12 months of drilling span two calendar years, you get two small write-offs instead of one big one. So if you know you'll need to shelter a lot of income in a particular calendar year, invest in a drilling program that starts in January or February.

If you invest in a successful drilling program, you may be assessed extra funds—typically, 10 to 30 percent of your original stake. It's natural to react to such assessments, more accurately termed overcalls, with anger, but you'd be wise to pay; in fact, the general partner may insist on it. Usually the additional money is used to drill "gravy wells"—because the first well proved so productive that geologists are sure of finding another gusher next door. And don't forget that most of the assessment will be deductible as intangible expense.

Once a well goes into production—is completed—its oil and/or gas reserves are estimated and a liquidating value—the amount you can sell your share for—is established. The liquidating value may discount the actual value of your share by as much as 70 to 80 percent. It's periodically updated to reflect depletion of reserves and other factors. Since you invested in order to shelter your income from taxes, it's to your advantage to sell out as soon as possible after the first year—usually in two to four years, depending on the rate of return you realize. If you like investing in oil and gas, the price you get for your share of that first well will finance your investment in a second well, with another big first-year write-off.

Because they lack an underlying hard asset, oil and gas investments are spared the problems of overvaluation associated with investments in real estate and equipment leasing. Their problem is more likely to be creative bookkeeping, something that only an accountant's audit could be expected to uncover.

There is another possible shortcoming that financial advisers like to warn of: It is estimated that only a quarter of the oil and gas tax-shelter packages offered publicly will ever serve you better than staid municipal bonds.

But if you're at the point where you feel you must try to find a shelter potentially more rewarding than municipals, don't despair. There still are plenty of them around. Just remember that there are caveats to be honored—and the need to sidestep so-called abusive shelters should be considered foremost among them.

"Ironically," says Roxanne Coady, an accountant with the national firm of Seidman and Seidman, "tax shelters on the whole are better investments than ever before. All the new rules have forced promoters to put the economics back into them."

Further reading 10

Further reading 10

This little book was intended primarily as an introduction to the fascinating—and potentially profitable—world of investing. If it has piqued your interest, you'll want to read more. And if it has led you to a decision that you want to move seriously into investments, you must read more.

For news of companies, industries, and the economic climate, look first to your daily newspaper. For greater depth in those areas, you'll want to subscribe to *The Wall Street Journal* and perhaps a specialized weekly such as *Barron's*. If stocks, bonds, and mutual funds are to become your major investment vehicles, you'll want to keep Standard & Poor's monthly *Stock Guide*, and possibly the S&P *Bond Guide*, readily available for easy reference.

Keeping up with the specific types of investments you find most appealing becomes essential once you've established an investment program. That could entail subscribing to one or more newsletters of the type we list here, at least some of which you should be able to sample at your broker's office.

And to satisfy your developed appetite for general investment information, there's no shortage of books. Those we list here, some containing advice that transcends the years, may suggest starters for a basic financial library. But once you've developed specific investment interests, you'll do well to spend a little time browsing through library card files and brokers' reference shelves for reading materials that satisfy them.

NEWSLETTERS AND ADVISORY SERVICES

Babson's Reports Investment & Barometer Letter, Wellesley Hills, Ma. 02181. Published weekly, $96 a year. This newsletter reviews major industries and factors affecting them, and selects and analyzes key stocks. Also provides an overview of the market and world events.

Indicator Digest, 451 Grand Ave., Palisades Park, N.J. 07650. Published 24 times a year, $125 a year. Somewhat more sophisticated but highly readable, it analyzes fundamental and technical factors to rate industry groups and draw conclusions on broad market strength. The *Digest* also includes articles on economic and market trends, coverage of bonds and government obligations, and follow-ups to previous recommendations.

Investor's Tax Shelter Report, 223 Duke of Gloucester St., Annapolis, Md. 21401. Published monthly, $125 a year. Provides in-depth and authoritative articles about all aspects of oil-and-gas investments, as well as monthly ratings of major publicly offered oil-and-gas tax shelters. Worthwhile for the serious oil-and-gas investor.

Real Estate Investing Letter, 757 Third Ave., New York, N.Y. 10017. Published monthly, $72 a year. Gives valuable how-to information for the real-estate investor, even the small-timer. Includes a section on the latest real-estate trends.

Research Institute Recommendations, 589 Fifth Ave., New York, N.Y. 10017. Published monthly, $48 a year. Contains wide-ranging information on developments affecting investments of all kinds and provides explanations of tax-law changes pertaining to investments.

Standard & Poor's *Outlook*, 25 Broadway, New York, N.Y. 10004. Published weekly, $175 a year. A cover-page summary of the contents helps the new investor through the charts and statistics inside. Provides a regular review of stock performance. Also from Standard & Poor's: two monthly publications, *Stock Guide* and *Bond Guide*, which provide detailed information on virtually every issue. Unless you're an extremely active investor, check your broker's copy.

United Business & Investment Report, 210 Newbury St., Boston, Ma. 02116. Published weekly, $170 a year. Easily understood coverage of a wide range of investment areas, with forthright recommendations on specific stocks and analyses of trends in the economy.

United Mutual Fund Selector, same address as above. Published semimonthly, $75 a year. An instructive, highly readable presentation of performance of funds and new developments in the field.

The Value Line Investment Survey, 711 Third Ave., New York, N.Y. 10017. Published weekly, $365 a year. Designed for completeness rather than easy reading and generally for the more sophisticated investor, this publication rates stocks by quality, yield, and long-term and short-term growth possibilities.

BOOKS

Investments: An Introduction to Analysis and Management, 4th ed, by Frederick Amling. Prentice-Hall, 1978, $21.00. Excellent textbook.

The New Options Market, rev ed, by Max G. Ansbacher. Walker & Co., 1979, $16.95. Easy to read and use.

Handbook of Wealth Management, by Leo Barnes and Stephen Feldman. McGraw-Hill, 1977, $42.50. Compendium of financial information.

Follow the Leaders, by Richard Blackman. Cornerstone Library (division of Simon & Schuster), 1979, $3.95. One of the best.

Winning: The Psychology of Successful Investing, by Srully Blotnick. McGraw-Hill, 1978, $15.95. Interesting, informative, verbose.

The Dow Jones-Irwin Guide to Put and Call Options, rev ed, by Henry Clasing. Dow Jones-Irwin, 1978, $14.95. Solid textbook.

The Dowbeaters: How to Buy Stocks That Go Up, by Ira Cobleigh and Bruce Dorfman. Macmillan, 1979, $10.95. For fun more than for profit.

Guide to Intelligent Investing, edited by Jerome B. Cohen. Dow Jones-Irwin, 1978, $12.50. A basic book, helpful for everyone.

The Sophisticated Investor, rev ed, by Burton Crane. Simon & Schuster, 1964, $2.95. Old but good.

Stock Market Strategy, by Richard A. Crowell. McGraw-Hill, 1977, $21.95. Solid background by a seasoned professional.

Investment Analysis and Management, by Anthony J. Curley and Robert M. Bear. Harper & Row, 1979, $24.50. For serious investors only.

The Complete Bond Book: A Guide to All Types of Fixed-Income Securities, by David M. Darst. McGraw-Hill, 1975, $22.50. Solid, comprehensive advice with plenty of simplified formulas, worksheets, charts, and tables.

Heads You Win, Tails You Win, by Ray Dirks. Stein & Day, 1979, $10.95. Light and lively.

Technical Analysis of Stock Trends, 5th ed, by Robert D. Edwards and John Magee. John Magee Associates, $45.00. Essential for serious traders.

How to Buy Stocks, 6th rev ed, by Louis Engel and Peter Wyckoff. Bantam, 1977, $3.50. A classic.

Dow Jones Investors Handbook, edited by Maurice Farrell. Dow Jones-Irwin, 1980, $5.95. A mighty tome for reference.

The Stock Options Manual, 2nd ed, by Gary L. Gastineau. McGraw-Hill, 1978, $18.95. All you ever need to know about options.

The Intelligent Investor: A Book of Practical Counsel, 4th rev ed, by Benjamin Graham. Harper & Row, 1973, $12.95. Old but good.

Security Analysis, 4th ed, by Benjamin Graham et al. McGraw-Hill, 1962, $22.50. Erudite, thoughtful, useful.

The Dow Jones-Irwin Guide to Modern Portfolio Theory, by Robert Hagin. Dow Jones-Irwin, 1980, $14.50. Best for professionals.

Dun & Bradstreet's Guide to Your Investments, by C. Colburn Hardy. Harper & Row, 1982, $16.75. Fact-packed with lists, tables, charts, and sample portfolios.

The Investor's Guide to Technical Analysis, by C. Colburn Hardy. McGraw-Hill, 1978, $15.95. All the amateur needs to know.

The Great American Bond Market: Selected Speeches of Sidney Homer, by Sidney Homer. Dow Jones-Irwin, 1978, $17.50. The bible of fixed-income investing.

The Battle for Investment Survival, rev ed, by Gerald M. Loeb. Simon & Schuster, 1965, $2.45. A basic book with insights from the late broker whose successes have become legendary.

A Random Walk Down Wall Street, rev ed, by Burton Malkiel. Norton, 1973, $13.95. Easy to take.

Tax Shelters That Work for Everyone: A Common Sense Guide to Keeping More of the Money You Earn, by Judith McQuown. McGraw-Hill, 1979, $12.95. Good basic guide, but tax information needs updating.

Real Estate Principles and Practices, 9th ed, by Alfred A. Ring and Jerome Dasso. Prentice-Hall, 1981, $26.50. Classic textbook in the field.

Real Estate Investment Strategies, 2nd ed, by Maury Seldin and Richard H. Swesnik. Wiley, 1979, $19.00. Basic, easy to understand.

The Thinking Investor's Guide to the Stock Market, by Kiril Sokoloff. McGraw-Hill, 1978, $15.95. A highly readable analysis.

Moneypower: How to Profit From Inflation, by Ben and Herbert Stein. Harper & Row, 1980, $8.95. Light and lively.

The Money Market: Myth, Reality and Practice, by Marcia Stigum. Dow Jones-Irwin, 1978, $27.50. All you need to know about money-market funds . . . and more.

The Money Masters: Nine Great Investors, Their Winning Strategies and How You Can Apply Them, by John Train. Harper & Row, 1980, $11.95. Better for personal pleasure than for financial information.

The Aggressive Conservative Investor, by Martin Whitman and Martin Shubik. Random House, 1979, $15.95. Good for checking ideas.

INDEX

A
Accelerated cost recovery system (ACRS), 82-83, *84*, 85, 114, 115, 119, *121*
Advisory services and newsletters, 129-130
American Stock Exchange (ASE; Amex), 13, 17

B
Babson, David L. & Co. Inc., *19-20*, 23
Bankers' acceptances, 59-60, *68-69*
Barron's, 13, *68*, 128
Bearer bonds, 27
"Big Board." See New York Stock Exchange
Bonds
  bearer, 27
  callable, 27, 28, 37, 40
  discounted, 28-29, 34
  growth, 28
  income, 34
  market price, 28-29
  mutual funds, 36
  "point," 29
  safety of principal, 32-34
  "senior" securities, 27
  trusts, 36
  yield, 26, 29, *30-31*
Broker
  bonds, 31, 32
  commission, 31
  real estate, 75, 77, 80
  stocks. See Stockbroker
Bull market, 19, 22, 59, 90

Page numbers in italics refer to boxed items.

C
Callable bonds, 27, 28, 37, 40
Call options, 92-93
Call protection, 28, 40
Capital gains
  bonds and, 29
  leased equipment, sale of, 122
  long-term, 8, 77
  rationale for investment, 7
  real estate, 74, 79, 82, 83, 115
  tax, 7, 8, 74, 79, 82, 83, 115
"Cash equivalents," 59
Certificates of deposit (CDs), 60
  comparison with T-bills, 61-62
  features, listing of, *66-67*
  maturity, 60
  premature withdrawal, 62
  six-month, 63-65
Certified commercial-investment member (CCIM), Realtors National Marketing Institute, 75
Chicago Board Options Exchange, 92, 93
Closed-end funds, 51
Commercial paper, 60, *68-69*
Commodity futures, 93-95
Convertibles ("CV"), 40-41
Corporate bond funds, 47, *49*
Corporate bonds, 33
Coupon rate, 29, *30*
Coupons, 27, *30*

D
Debentures, 33
Depletion allowance, 124, 125
Depreciation
  accelerated cost recovery system (ACRS), 82-83, *84*, 85, 114-115, 119, *121*

declining-balance, 82-83
equipment leasing, 118-119, 121-122
land, 82
real estate, 76-77, 78, 81-83, 84, 85
recapture, 82, 83, 85, 114-116, 119, *121*, 122
straight-line, 76-77, 82, 83, 85, 114-115, 119, *120*
sum-of-years-digits, 119
Discount brokerage houses, 15-16, 31
Diversification, 18, 36, 45
Dividends
  common-stock, 11
  fixed, 11
  growth funds, 47
  growth-stock, 7, 9
  growth-with-income funds, 47
  income funds, 47
  money-market funds, 50
  performance funds, 47
  preferred stocks, 11
  undeclared, 27
Dow Jones Industrial Average (DJIA) *14*, 19, 22

E

Earnings
  per-share, 9-10
  progression of increase, 10
Economic Recovery Tax Act of 1981
  energy exploration and, 123
  equipment leasing and, 118, 121
  real estate revisions, 85, 114
  tax shelters and, 98
End-of-the-lease purchase agreement, 118
Energy exploration and development
  depletion allowance, 124
  investment tax credit, 124-125

windfall-profits tax, 123-124
Equipment leasing
  depreciation, 118-119
  end-of-the-lease purchase agreement, 118
  fast write-off, 118-119
  investment tax credit, 119-120
  tax treatment according to class, *120-121*
Escalation clause, 79

F

Fast write-off, 118-119
Federal Home Loan Bank Board, 33
Federal National Mortgage Association, 33
Federal Reserve, Treasury bills, *62-63*
Federal Reserve bank(s), 61, *62-63*
Federal Reserve board, 90
Foreclosure, 116-117

G

Gas drilling. See Energy exploration and development
Growth funds, 47, *48*
Growth mutual funds, *52-55*
Growth stocks, 7-9
  portfolio sample, *19-21*
Growth-with-income funds, 47, *48*

I

Income, unearned, 7-8, 117
Income funds, 47, *48-49*
Income stocks
  portfolio sample, *19-21*
  yield, 7-9
Individual Retirement Accounts (IRAs), 54, 99, 100
Interest
  equipment leasing, 122
  margin accounts, 89-90
  mortgage, 74, 75, 76, 78

municipal short-term notes, 66-67
Treasury bills, 32-33, 61-62, 66-67
U.S. agency short-term notes, 66-67
Interest rates
  bonds and, 26, 27, 28, 29, *30-31*, 34, 40
  certificates of deposit, 60, 66-67, 70
  money-market mutual funds, 69-70
  money markets and, 58-59
  savings accounts, 66-67
  stock market, effect on, 59
  Treasury bills, 32, 70
Internal Revenue Service (IRS)
  investment tax credits and, 119
  real estate depreciation and, 74, 76, 78, 81-83, 84, 85, 114-116
  tax shelters and, 100, 103, 107, 110-112, 113-117
Investment diversification. *See* Portfolio, diversification of
Investment-letter stock. *See* Letter stock
Investment objectives, 7-9, 32-36, 46
Investment tax credit
  energy exploration, 123-125
  equipment leasing, 119, *120-121*, 122
  exotic tax shelters, 107-108
  limits, 119-120, 122
  recapture, *121*
IRS. *See* Internal Revenue Service

J
Joint venture, 124

L
Lasser, J.K., *Your Income Tax*, 75

Letter stock, 91-92
Leverage, 77, 89, 94
Limited partnerships
  energy exploration and, 124
  investment tax credit, 119-122
  real estate and, 79-80, 112-117
  tax shelter and, 99, 101, 106, 112-117
Lipper Analytical Services Inc., 51
Liquidating value, energy exploration, 126
Load funds, 46, 51, *54-55*

M
Margin accounts, 88-90
Merrill Lynch, Pierce, Fenner & Smith Inc., 15, *16*, 94, 98
Money market. *See also* Money-market funds
  bankers' acceptances, 59-60, 68-69
  certificates, 63-65
  certificates of deposit, 60, 66-67
  commercial paper, 60, 68-69
  minimum investment, 58, 59
  mutual funds, 18, *49*, 50, 54, 58, 59, 68-70
  Treasury bills, 60-62, 66-67
  U.S. agency short-term notes, 66-67
Money-market certificates, 63-65
Money-market funds, 18, 50, 54, 70
  dividends, 50
  interest rates and, 69-70
  list of, *49*, *64-65*
  minimum initial investment, 50, *64-65*, 68
  operating expenses, 69
  types of investments, 50
  withdrawal, 68
  yields, 50, 68-70
Moody's Investors Service Inc.

Index   137

bond ratings, 33
reference materials, 13, 36
Mortgage(s)
 bonds, 33
 interest on, 74, 78
 purchase-money, 75-76
Municipal-bond funds, 47, 49, 50
Municipal bonds ("munis")
 purchasing of, 32
 tax advantage, 35, *37-39*
 as tax shelter, 99-100
 yields, 35, *37-39*
Municipal bond trusts, 47, 50
Municipal short-term notes, 66-67
Mutual funds
 advantages, 44-46
 bond, 36
 closed-end, 51
 corporate-bond, 47, *49*
 fees, management and operating, 46
 growth, 47, *48, 52-54*
 growth-with-income, 47, *48*
 income, 47, *48-49*
 listing, *48-49, 52-53, 54-55*
 load, 46, *54-55*
 money-market, *49*, 50, 58, 68-70
 municipal-bond, 47, *49*, 50
 no-load, 46, *52-53*, 54
 open-end, 51
 performance, 47, *48*
 selection of, 50-51, 54-55
 types of, 47, 50

N

National Association of Real Estate Investment Trusts (NAREIT), 80
National Association of Securities Dealers, 12
Newsletters and advisory services, 129-130
New York Stock Exchange (NYSE; Big Board), 12, *14*, 17

No-load funds, 46, *52-53*, 54
Non-callable (N/C) bonds, 37, 40
Nonrecourse loan, 114, 115, 116, 119-120

O

Odd lot, 17
Oil drilling. *See* Energy exploration and development
Open-end fund, 51
Option trading, 92-93
Overcalls, 125
Over-the-counter (OTC) market, 13, 80

P

Par value, 29, *30-31*
Performance funds, 47, *48*
Per-share earnings, 9
Physicians
 real estate investments favored, *73*
 tax shelter solicitation and, 102-104
Portfolio
 balancing with income stocks, 9
 bond features and, 30
 diversification of, 18-19, 36, 45
 "mix," 26
 samples of, *19-21*
 self-management, 15
Preferred stocks, 11-12, 47
Price-to-earnings (P/E) ratio, 10-11, *15*, *21*
Prospectus
 energy exploration, 125
 limited partnership, real estate, 80
 mutual funds, 46, 51, 54
 tax shelters, 100, 106-107
Public offerings, 113
Put and call options, 92-93

Q

Quick & Reilly, 16

R

Real-estate investment
  commercial property, 72, 73, 83, 85, 114
  depreciation, 74, 76, 78-79, 81-83, 84, 85, 114-116
  farm acreage, 72, 73
  information sources, 74-75
  leverage, 77
  limited partnerships, 79-80, 112-117
  location, 75-76, 78, 81
  nonrecourse loan, 114, 115, 116
  rental housing, 72, 73
  residential property, 75-77, 83, 115
  sale-and-leaseback, 78-79
  taxes, 74-77
  tax shelters, 78, 79, 112-118
  triple-net lease, 79
  undeveloped land (raw land), 72, 73, 81
Real-estate investment trusts (REITs), 79, 80
Realtors National Marketing Institute, 75
Recapture
  avoidance, 122
  defined, 82, 83
  equipment depreciation, 119, 121, 122
  investment tax credit, 121
  real estate depreciation, 82, 83, 85, 114-116
Recourse loan, 108
Registered bonds, 27
REITs. See Real-estate investment trusts
REITs Quarterly, 80
Retirement plan, mutual funds in, 54
Round lot, 17

S

Sale-and-leaseback, 78-79
Salomon Brothers, 68
Savings accounts, 66-67
Savings certificates. See Money-market certificates
Securities and Exchange Commission (SEC)
  interstate regulation and, 32
  limited partnership registration, 106
  registration of corporations, 36, 46, 91
Selling short, 90-91
Short-term investments. See also Bankers' acceptances; Certificates of deposit; Commercial paper; Money-market certificates; Money-market funds; Municipal short-term notes; Savings accounts; Treasury bills; U.S. agency short-term notes
  list of, 66-69
  yields, 66, 68, 69, 70
Speculators, 93-94
Standard & Poor's *Bond Guide*, 36, 128, 130
Standard & Poor's Corp., 14, 20, 54
  bond assessment, 33
  reference material, 13, 36, 51, 128, 130
Standard & Poor's *Outlook*, 130
Standard & Poor's *Stock Guide*, 51, 128, 130
Stock(s)
  characteristics of high-quality, 19-21
  common, 11-13, 14
  comparison with bonds, 26
  dividends, 7-8, 9, 15, 19, 21
  "equity" issues, 26
  growth, 7-9, 19-21
  income, 7-9, 19-21
  letter, 91-92
  listed, 12
  margin accounts, 88-90

measurement of relative worth, 9-11, *14-15*
option trading, 92-93
portfolio, 18, *19-21*
preferred, 11-12, 47
prices, 9-11, *14-15*, *21*, 83-85
purchasing of, 17-18, 23
registration, 91-92
selling short, 90-91
splits, 7, 17
trading range, *14*
trading volume, *15*
unlisted, 12
unregistered, 91
yield, 7, 8, *15*, *19-21*

Stockbroker
 bonds and, 31-32
 choosing, 13-16
 commissions, 15-16, 31-32
 mutual funds and, 54

Stock-brokerage firms
 discount, 15-16, 31
 full-service, 14-16
 leading, *16*

Stock market
 American Stock Exchange, 13, 17
 breadth indices, *15*
 investment decisions, 6
 New York Stock Exchange, 12, *14*, 17
 over-the-counter, 13, 80
 real-estate investment trusts, 80
 report, *14-15*
 trends, *14-15*, 22-23

Stock market report, *14-15*
Stock splits, 7, 17
Street name, 18

T

Tax(es)
 bonds and, 26, 32-33, 35-36, *37-39*
 capital gains, 7, 8, 74, 77
 credits. See Investment tax credit
 deduction. See Tax deductions
 deferred, 99-100
 Economic Recovery Tax Act of 1981, 85, 98, 114, 118, 123
 energy exploration and development, 123-126
 equipment leasing, 118-123
 government-agency bonds, 32-33
 ordinary income, 85
 real-estate investments, 74, 83, 85, 113-117
 savings, 30, 34, 112, 114-115, 122
 shelters. See Tax shelters
 Treasury bills, 33, 61, 67
 unearned income, 7, 8, 98, 117
 windfall-profits, 123-124

Tax bracket
 equipment leasing and, 121
 income stocks and, 8-9
 municipal bonds and, 35, *37-39*
 real-estate investment and, 77, 114
 tax shelters and, 102, 112

Tax deductions
 depreciation, 74, 76-77, 78, 81-83, 84, 85, 114-115, 121-122
 energy exploration, 125, 126
 equipment, 121
 interest, 74, 78, 115, 122
 professional management, 79

Tax laws
 Economic Recovery Tax Act of 1981, 85, 98, 114, 118, 123
 energy exploration and, 123-124
 equipment leasing and, 118
 real-estate investments and, 83, 85, 113-115

Revenue Act of 1978, 111
Tax Equity and Fiscal
    Responsibility Act of
    1982, 111
Tax Reduction Act of 1975,
    111
Tax Reform Act of 1969, 111
    tax shelters and, 111
Windfall Profit Tax Act of
    1980, 111
Tax shelter(s)
    abuses, 111-112
    disallowed, 100
    energy exploration, 123-126
    equipment leasing, 118-123
    exotic, 95, 107-108, 123
    investor considerations, 101-
        102
    limited partnership, 99, 112-
        118
    liquidity, 101
    real estate, 78-79, 112-118
    solicitation, 102-104
T-bills. See Treasury bills
Thrift certificates. See Money-
    market certificates
Treasuries, 32-33
Treasury bills
    coupon yield, 61
    features, listing of, 66-67
    minimum investment, 33, 60,
        66
    purchasing of, 60-61, 62-63
Treasury bonds, 32, 61
Treasury notes, 33, 61
Triple-net lease, 79

Trusts
    bond, 36
    municipal-bond, 47, 50

U
*United Business & Investment
    Report*, 48, 130
United Business Service, 51
U.S. agency short-term notes,
    66-67
U.S. Master Tax Guide, 74-75

V
*Value Line Investment Survey,
    The*, 13, 130

W
Wall Street Journal, The, 12, 68,
    69, 107, 128
Wiesenberger Investment
    Companies Service, 51, 54
Windfall-profits tax, 123-124

Y
Yield
    bond, 26, 29, *30-31*
    coupon, 61
    fixed, 26, 29
    growth stock, 7, 8, *19-21*
    income funds, 47
    income stock, 8, *19-21*
    money-market certificates,
        63-65
    money-market funds, 50, 68-
        70
    money-market instruments,
        66-69
    municipal-bond funds, 47
    municipal bonds, 35, *37-39*
    taxable versus tax-free, *37-39*
    to maturity, calculating, *30-31*
Your Income Tax (Lasser), 75

Other Titles of Related Interest From Medical Economics Books

**ABCs of Investing Your Retirement Funds
Second Edition**
   C. Colburn Hardy
   ISBN 0-87489-259-7

Tax Strategy for Physicians, Second Edition
   Lawrence Farber
   ISBN 0-87489-258-9

Insurance Strategies for Physicians
   Phillips Huston
   ISBN 0-87489-279-1

**Personal Pension Plan Strategies
for Physicians**
   C. Colburn Hardy
   ISBN 0-87489-345-3

**Personal Money Management for Physicians
Third Edition**
   Lawrence Farber, Editor
   ISBN 0-87489-253-8

**Computerizing Your Medical Office:
A Guide for Physicians and Their Staffs**
   Dot Sellars
   ISBN 0-87489-305-4

**Designing and Building Your Own
Professional Office**
   Murray Schwartz, D.D.S.
   ISBN 0-87489-228-7

**How to Buy or Sell Your Home
in a Changing Market**
   Warren Boroson
   ISBN 0-87489-278-3

Revenue Act of 1978, 111
Tax Equity and Fiscal
  Responsibility Act of
  1982, 111
Tax Reduction Act of 1975,
  111
Tax Reform Act of 1969, 111
  tax shelters and, 111
Windfall Profit Tax Act of
  1980, 111
Tax shelter(s)
  abuses, 111-112
  disallowed, 100
  energy exploration, 123-126
  equipment leasing, 118-123
  exotic, 95, 107-108, 123
  investor considerations, 101-102
  limited partnership, 99, 112-118
  liquidity, 101
  real estate, 78-79, 112-118
  solicitation, 102-104
T-bills. See Treasury bills
Thrift certificates. See Money-market certificates
Treasuries, 32-33
Treasury bills
  coupon yield, 61
  features, listing of, 66-67
  minimum investment, 33, 60, 66
  purchasing of, 60-61, 62-63
Treasury bonds, 32, 61
Treasury notes, 33, 61
Triple-net lease, 79

Trusts
  bond, 36
  municipal-bond, 47, 50
U
United Business & Investment
  Report, 48, 130
United Business Service, 51
U.S. agency short-term notes,
  66-67
U.S. Master Tax Guide, 74-75
V
Value Line Investment Survey,
  The, 13, 130
W
Wall Street Journal, The, 12, 68,
  69, 107, 128
Wiesenberger Investment
  Companies Service, 51, 54
Windfall-profits tax, 123-124
Y
Yield
  bond, 26, 29, 30-31
  coupon, 61
  fixed, 26, 29
  growth stock, 7, 8, 19-21
  income funds, 47
  income stock, 8, 19-21
  money-market certificates,
    63-65
  money-market funds, 50, 68-70
  money-market instruments,
    66-69
  municipal-bond funds, 47
  municipal bonds, 35, 37-39
  taxable versus tax-free, 37-39
  to maturity, calculating, 30-31
Your Income Tax (Lasser), 75

Other Titles of Related Interest From Medical Economics Books

ABCs of Investing Your Retirement Funds
Second Edition
C. Colburn Hardy
ISBN 0-87489-259-7

Tax Strategy for Physicians, Second Edition
Lawrence Farber
ISBN 0-87489-258-9

Insurance Strategies for Physicians
Phillips Huston
ISBN 0-87489-279-1

Personal Pension Plan Strategies for Physicians
C. Colburn Hardy
ISBN 0-87489-345-3

Personal Money Management for Physicians
Third Edition
Lawrence Farber, Editor
ISBN 0-87489-253-8

Computerizing Your Medical Office: A Guide for Physicians and Their Staffs
Dot Sellars
ISBN 0-87489-305-4

Designing and Building Your Own Professional Office
Murray Schwartz, D.D.S.
ISBN 0-87489-228-7

How to Buy or Sell Your Home in a Changing Market
Warren Boroson
ISBN 0-87489-278-3

Medical Practice Management, Revised Edition
  Horace Cotton
  ISBN 0-87489-098-5

How to Hire, Train, and Manage Your Employees
  Marianne Dekker Mattera, Editor
  ISBN 0-87489-270-8

How to Close a Medical Practice
  Gene Balliett
  ISBN 0-87489-142-6

The Whys and Wherefores of Corporate Practice Fourth Edition
  Sheldon H. Gorlick, J.D.
  ISBN 0-87489-264-3

Now That You've Incorporated, Fourth Edition Coping With Changing Tax Laws
  Sheldon H. Gorlick, J.D.
  ISBN 0-87489-272-4

Testifying in Court, Second Edition
  Jack E. Horsley, J.D., and John Carlova
  ISBN 0-87489-315-1

Medical Economics Encyclopedia of Practice and Financial Management
  Edited by Lawrence Farber
  ISBN 0-87489-343-7

For information, write to:

Medical Economics Books
Oradell, New Jersey 07649
Or call toll-free: 1-800-223-0581, ext. 2755
(Within the 201 area: 262-3030, ext. 2755)

HETERICK MEMORIAL LIBRARY
332.678 H324b 1984   onuu
Harsham, Philip/The beginning investor

3 5111 00158 6803